STO

DO NOT REMOVE
CARDS FROM POCKET

Primary Medical Care
of Children and Adolescents

Primary Medical Care of Children and Adolescents

William Feldman
Walter Rosser
Patrick McGrath

New York   Oxford
OXFORD UNIVERSITY PRESS
1987

Oxford University Press

Oxford   New York   Toronto
Delhi   Bombay   Calcutta   Madras   Karachi
Petaling Jaya   Singapore   Hong Kong   Tokyo
Nairobi   Dar es Salaam   Cape Town
Melbourne   Auckland
and associated companies in
Beirut   Berlin   Ibadan   Nicosia

Published by Oxford University Press, Inc.,
200 Madison Avenue, New York, New York 10016

Oxford is a registered trademark of Oxford University Press

Library of Congress Cataloging-in-Publication Data

Feldman, William.
    Primary medical care of children and adolescents.
    Includes bibliographies and index.
    1. Pediatrics.   2. Adolescent medicine.   3. Family medicine.
I. Rosser, Walter.   II. McGrath, Patrick J.   III. Title.
[DNLM: 1. Adolescent medicine.   2. Pediatrics.
3. Primary Health Care.   WS 100 F312p]
RJ47.F45   1987   618.92   86–28566
ISBN 0–19–504298–0

10 9 8 7 6 5 4 3 2 1

Printed in the United States of America

FOREWORD

Although most medical textbooks do not have a foreword, this one is sufficiently different in its perspective to warrant a few comments from a long-time observer of the passing scene in medical education. For some two generations, textbooks on clinical subjects have been written from the viewpoint of the hospital-based tertiary care super-specialist. Though clearly important, this viewpoint is not the only one, nor does it encompass the vast bulk of medical problems experienced by most people most of the time. Nor is it the viewpoint from which the clinicians who manage these initial problems approach them or their patients.

The authors of most clinical textbooks are constrained by the selective bias associated with the undeniable need to provide appropriate tertiary care for that relatively small subset of clinical problems seen in university hospitals and major medical centers. By definition this subset consists largely of rare, unusually complicated conditions or those requiring complex or expensive equipment. This level of care calls for clinicians who are narrowly focussed and highly specialized. As a consequence, few of them have opportunities to observe the complete natural history of those problems in which they do specialize. And although these truncated encounters bring obvious benefits, few will argue that most tertiary care super-specialists experience the full diversity of health problems which beset the general population. The super-specialist's experience is constricted both vertically and horizontally. And that is not all.

The contemporary context in which most tertiary care is conducted usually employs a reductionist, deterministic and mono-etiological paradigm. This largely outmoded model of health and disease tends to exclude consideration of psychological and behavioral components in either the genesis of or the response to illness. To distort matters further, the object of the exercise for many super-specialists is usually much less to manage the patient's problem effectively and expeditiously than to embark on an exhaustive, and sometimes mindless, search for rare conditions of low probability for which there is often little or no efficacious treatment. "Rule out" and "must not miss" become the operative guidelines, and "diagnosis" becomes an end in itself rather than a label or "code word" that serves to guide demonstrably efficacious interventions.

As a consequence, textbooks based on tertiary care experience alone are of limited value, except as reference books, to those serving at the coal-face of primary medical care, i.e., the family physicians, general practitioners, general internists, and general pediatricians who provide the great bulk of medical care in the western world.

The net effect of the narrow perspective characterizing most clinical textbooks has been to give an unbalanced view of medical practice and research to both undergraduate and postgraduate students. In turn, these institutional imbalances are reflected in the content of medical education and clinical experience at all levels. The academic environment that results has far-reaching negative perturbations which influence the attitudes, knowledge, priorities, and skills made available to the public by the collective medical establishment. The dominance of the "top-down," tertiary care view of medicine's task is apparent in the absurd imbalances that persist in the allocation of resources and provision of health services and the seemingly endless increases in the overall costs of medical care. Nor are matters helped by the control of research funds by those who have had little exposure to the population-based perspective. As a consequence, research at the level of primary care is seriously neglected and, in turn, the curiosity of both students and faculty in these problems lies fallow.

Primary medical care is now recognized as the basic and, indeed, by far the major component of any rationally arranged health care system. Exemplary primary medical care, equitably available to all, is needed universally for the provision of preventive services, as well as for health education and health promotion through counselling during the "teachable moment." But, of equal importance, primary medical care is essential for early management of illnesses of all types, for keeping people out of hospitals if possible, and for referring them promptly to sources of tertiary care when necessary. If all this were not enough, primary medical care is a sine qua non for containing costs.

To provide exemplary primary medical care, family physicians, general internists, and general pediatricians employ a probabilistic approach to understanding their patients' problems. Usually this approach is appropriate when there is ample time to observe the course of the patient's distress or illness, to gather further data or evidence, to test hypotheses or to evaluate the outcome of interventions. Accomplishing all this, however, requires a different perspective and different kinds of information from those currently available in most clinical textbooks. A probabilistic orientation, a multi-causal, nonlinear paradigm, and a hypothesis-testing approach to clinical management are the essential ingredients.

This volume must surely be a first. As such, perhaps it heralds a new generation of population-based, problem-oriented textbooks that start with the patient and the problem the clinician encounters. An epidemiological or population-based perspective is evident throughout the volume. Common problems are recognized as "common" and rare conditions as "rare"! The clinician is encouraged to think about the most likely condition first and to employ a probabilistic, nonlinear approach to gathering information and testing hypotheses. The existence of serious treatable diseases is recognized as well as the need for prompt and appropriate referral for consultation.

Another "first" for this pioneering textbook is the assignment of levels of credibility to the evidence supporting most of the interventions discussed. It is still unusual to find a complete textbook of internal medicine or pediatrics that evaluates the relative efficacy of all the treatments recommended. Use of the terms "No Clear Evidence," "Suggestive Evidence," and "Firm Evidence" to designate the likelihood that a specific intervention will do more good than harm must surely enhance the physician's clinical skills and overall capacities to serve the population. The introduction in a clinical textbook of "critical appraisal" techniques based on epidemiological principles is long overdue.

In summary, *Primary Medical Care of Children and Adolescents* establishes a new format and new objectives for clinical textbooks in medicine. By using epidemiological perspectives, the authors encourage a probabilistic and population-based approach to understanding patients' problems and by using epidemiological methods for critical appraisal of evidence they classify the relative efficacy of various interventions. What has been done for children in this volume could surely be done for adults at the level of primary care, and there is every reason to look forward to future specialized textbooks being organized along similar lines.

I hope medical students, as well as house officers and practitioners in family medicine, general pediatrics, and general internal medicine will learn much from this book. It should help them both to provide better care for their patients and to think more critically about the problems of health and disease in the populations they serve.

Stanardsville, Virginia   Kerr L. White, M.D.
August 1986

PREFACE

Most textbooks begin out of dissatisfaction, and this book is no exception. *Primary Medical Care of Children and Adolescents* grew from a desire to have a practical diagnostic and management guide to children's health problems encountered in primary care. We felt that such a book, unlike other available texts, should focus on the common problems that practitioners confront in their offices and the uncommon but important problems that may occasionally present. We considered a problem-oriented approach more appropriate than a systems-oriented one. We wanted a volume that would provide a scientific evaluation of the strength of evidence supporting suggested management strategies. We sought a book that would address problems that are primarily biological or primarily behavioral, as well as the many problems that have both biological and behavioral components. Unable to find a book that had more than one or two of these characteristics, we wrote *Primary Medical Care of Children and Adolescents*.

We have been careful not to develop yet another encyclopedic list of differential diagnoses or an exhaustive description of the diagnosis and treatment of the many rare problems that occur in children. There are several excellent pediatrics texts that meet this need (1,2). This book does not replace the standard pediatric textbooks, which should most appropriately be used as references for the unusual case or for exhaustive background on a problem.

We attempt to follow the clinical problem-solving techniques that primary care physicians actually use with a child patient. Barrows (3) has outlined the steps of the problem-solving process in primary care. The first step is to formulate an initial concept of what the problem is, for example, "an infant with a fever" or "an adolescent with weight problems." Subsequent steps simultaneously generate and investigate a number of competing hypotheses. Using multiple shortcuts based on the information gathered from the patient, the physician follows a problem-solving approach to narrow down the problem by eliminating options. For example, if the child with a fever is smiling, he is unlikely to have meningitis. The information is drawn primarily from the history and physical examination and to a much lesser extent from laboratory investigations. In the final steps, the physician arrives at a diagnosis and decides on management. The process is not a straightforward and linear one, but a dynamic, probabilistic process that is influenced by each bit of data given by the patient and by the physician's knowledge of the competing hypotheses. Although not linear, the process is logical.

The majority of the chapters follow a standard format that mimics the naturally occurring process described by Barrows. They are organized by problems that patients typically present with in the office. Each chapter opens with an introduction to the major subgroups of the problem, then, in the second section, gives prevalence data (if available). Each of the subproblems is narrowed down and a section on diagnosis follows. Finally, management of each problem is discussed, with a critical appraisal (with appropriate references) of the validity of management suggestions. The levels of quality of evidence are the same as the criteria of the Canadian Task Force on Periodic Health Examination, but we have used descriptive labels for each level. The levels of quality of evidence are NO CLEAR EVIDENCE; SUGGESTIVE EVIDENCE; and FIRM EVIDENCE. The criteria for the quality of evidence are contained in Table 1.

Slavish adherence to a predetermined model of the clinical problem-solving process in a book would require unnecessary detail and would overwhelm the reader with tedious information. Consequently, we have not used detailed algorithms but have opted for the frequent use of tables and a problem-solving style of presentation. Because of the nature of the material, some chapters, such as "Preventive Health Examination" (Chapter 14), do not follow our typical format. In all of the chapters we have attempted to use the types of shortcuts that clinicians actually use. Rare disorders are not given much attention unless they are discernible in primary care and have serious, preventable consequences. Common problems that are likely to be less well known to physicians are treated in more detail than topics likely to be well

Table 1. Quality of Evidence

Level	Description
NO CLEAR EVIDENCE	Opinions based on clinical experience, anecdotal case studies, or descriptive studies; conflicting evidence from studies or poorly designed studies, even if randomized, controlled trial
SUGGESTIVE EVIDENCE	Evidence from cohort, case control, correlational or replicated single-case experimental, pre-post studies
FIRM EVIDENCE	Evidence from at least one properly designed randomized, controlled trial considering sample selection, sample size, adequate controls, blinded, or clear reduction in mortality

known. For example, many of the common behavior problems that concern parents but for which primary care physicians have little training are discussed and referenced much more extensively than straightforward medical problems.

The chapters have been grouped into two sections: "Common Physical Problems in Primary Care" and "Growth, Development and Adaptation." The order of chapters within the sections roughly corresponds to the prevalence of the problems seen in practice.

We believe that *Primary Medical Care of Children and Adolescents* will be of use to family practitioners and primary care pediatricians, family practice and pediatric residents, medical students, nurse practitioners, and nursing students. Subspecialists probably will not like our treatment of their areas. We make no apology for this. We are writing for the primary care physician, not the person who has completed a subspeciality fellowship. We have purposely not included the detail that is necessary for the consultant but which, unfortunately, is frequently found in textbooks written by the consultant for generalists.

REFERENCES

1. Behrman, R.E., Vaughan, V.C., eds. *Nelson: Textbook of pediatrics.* 12th ed. Philadelphia: W. B. Saunders, 1983.
2. Rudolph, A.M., ed. *Pediatrics.* 17th ed. Norwalk, Conn.: Appleton-Century-Crofts, 1982.
3. Barrows, H.S., Tamblyn, R.M. *Problem-based learning: An approach to medical education.* New York: Springer, 1980.
4. Canadian Task Force on the Periodic Health Examination. *Can. Med. Assoc. J.* 121 (suppl.): 5, 1979.

ACKNOWLEDGMENTS

We wish to acknowledge the encouragement of the Children's Hospital of Eastern Ontario, the Ottawa Civic Hospital, and the University of Ottawa. We have been particularly privileged to work in departments where interdisciplinary endeavors are supported. The library staff at the Children's Hospital of Eastern Ontario was particularly helpful. Numerous colleagues have read and criticized the many versions of different chapters or assisted in various phases of finishing the manuscript. We wish to specifically thank L. Archer, M. Cornfield, J. Dunn-Geier, B. Feldman, J.T. Goodman, S. Kardash, J. L'Heureux, L. Levesque, I. Manion, I. McWhinney, R. Pilon, S. Pisterman, A. Schlieper, C. Serediuk, H. Tsun, and A. Unruh.

Although at different points each of us took primary responsibility for specific chapters, the book is the product of our joint, equal effort, and we share the blame for any errors or ommissions.

Dr. McGrath is supported by a Career Scientist Award of the Ontario Ministry of Health. Dr. Rosser moved from the Department of Family Medicine, University of Ottawa, to the Department of Family Medicine, McMaster University, as the book was being completed.

Thanks are due to our spouses for their patience and support.

Finally, the authors wish to thank the Poltimore Practical Pediatrics Group for stimulation, support, and guidance when it was unclear if this work would ever come to fruition.

Ontario   W. F.
July 1986   W. R.
                                                                                                             P. M.

CONTENTS

COMMON PHYSICAL PROBLEMS
IN PRIMARY CARE   1

GROWTH, DEVELOPMENT, AND ADAPTATION   127

Common Physical Problems
in Primary Care

1

FEVER

PREVALENCE

Fever (temperature greater than 38° C) and the illnesses associated with fever constitute the major reason that children are brought to a physician. For example, more than 90% of children have been infected with parainfluenza viruses by the age of 5 and almost 100% with respiratory syncytial virus by age 2; more than 60% of school-aged children have been infected with adenoviruses. Most of these illnesses are associated with respiratory symptoms and fever; many are self-limited.

Although the majority of febrile illnesses in infants and children are viral in origin and are associated with excellent outcomes, it is often difficult to distinguish the benign infections from those treatable bacterial infections that are life-threatening. The most prevalent illnesses resulting in fever in infants and children are respiratory infections, otitis media, and gastroenteritis. Serious, treatable bacterial infections, although not common, may cause death or disability if diagnosis is delayed. These illnesses include meningitis, pneumonia, urinary tract infections, osteomyelitis, and septicemia.

NARROWING DOWN

The common conditions associated with fever in infants and children are described in the chapters on upper respiratory (Chapter 2) and lower respiratory infections (Chapter 7), ear problems (Chapter 3), bowel problems (Chapter 5), and genitourinary problems (Chapter 10). The clinician's major goal is to separate obvious causes of fever with known treatments and prognoses from occult, potentially life-threatening illnesses. The diagnostic problems are most frequent in infants under 2 years of age, particularly in infants under 3 months of age. The major reasons for the difficulty in sorting out the benign from the sinister causes of fever in infants under 2 years are that these children cannot describe symptoms such as earache, dysuria, limb pain, or severe headache—clues to otitis media, urinary tract infection, osteomyelitis, or meningitis. In addition, signs such as neck stiffness, which are very predictive of meningitis in older children, are unreliable in young infants, who may have poor neck muscle tone. Thus the clinician's diagnostic tools of observation, physical examination, and judiciously chosen laboratory tests become even more important in this age group.

DIAGNOSIS

Infants 30 days of age or younger

Infants 30 days of age or younger are at risk of infection with group B beta-hemolytic streptococcus. This organism rarely produces significant effects in older infants. Meningitis or septicemia leading to fulminating shock and death may result from group B infections. Because young infants may show very few signs of illness other than fever early on, it has been recommended that they be managed differently from older infants not at risk from this bacterial agent. Although hospital admission, obtaining blood, urine and cerebrospinal fluid cultures and chest radiographs, and administering antibiotics have been recommended by some, there is NO CLEAR EVIDENCE that such an aggressive approach is required for all infants less than 30 days old. In fact, in one hospital where the policy is admission, a battery of tests, and antibiotics for all infants 2 months of age and under (1), only two-thirds of these babies were actually admitted, only 10% of those not admitted underwent the battery of tests, and all of those not admitted had excellent outcomes. The policy was most likely to be implemented for infants who were less than 30 days old with temperatures greater than 38.5°C. In another study, the number of admissions and the aggressiveness of investigations were inversely correlated with the level of clinical experience of the physician; the more senior physicians were considerably more selective in their approach (2).

Since serious infections in younger infants are more difficult to diagnose than those in older infants, it can be argued that an aggressive approach to diagnosis and treatment will improve mortality and morbidity in the few, and that this potential benefit outweighs the costs and risks for the many who would have excellent prognoses if not treated. The iatrogenic risks and financial costs of such an aggressive approach are not negligible. In one study, 20% of admissions resulted in complications such as skin sloughing at intravenous sites, aminoglycoside overdose, and nosocomial diarrhea. The average cost per admission was U.S. $2,130 (1979 dollars) (3).

In the absence of randomized, controlled trials, it is prudent to admit to the hospital infants less than 30 days old with fever and no focus of infection and to observe them in a holding unit or ward. Blood and urine cultures and a chest radiograph should be taken, and complete blood cell count (CBC) and erythrocyte sedimentation rate (ESR) determined. Lumbar puncture is not necessary for infants who remain clinically well for 24 hours. If the blood and urine cultures are negative, these infants will probably do well at home, without antibiotic treatment but with careful follow-up.

Infants between 1 and 3 months of age

Infants in the 1- to 3-month age group who have serious bacterial infections do not respond with an improved clinical appearance to antipyretic measures. Those who do look clinically well after antipyretic measures have been taken (see management), who have signs and symptoms of a viral upper respiratory infection, and whose family members have colds probably need no laboratory investigations. A period of observation in an outpatient setting will help determine if tests are required; for those who continue to look clinically well with no focal signs of infection, no combination of laboratory tests is as valuable as repeated follow-up. Follow-up can be done by telephone if the parents are reliable or by repeat clinical assessment if there are doubts.

Infants who continue to look ill after antipyretic measures have been taken should be treated in a manner similar to that for infants less than 1 month old because there is an increased risk of serious underlying bacterial infection. A lumbar puncture should be done if there is any suspicion of meningitis. Intravenous ampicillin (and chloramphenicol in 4 divided doses) should be administered pending the results of the CSF culture because of the risk of covert meningitis.

Infants 3 months to 2 years of age

The evidence regarding which laboratory tests should be done for febrile 3- to 24-month-olds is not based on randomized, controlled trials. The sensitivity (the ability to recognize those infants with occult life-threatening infections using various tests), and specificity (the ability to determine those with benign causes via normal test results) of a variety of laboratory tests are well known; their predictive value is questionable (4,5). What is more interesting is that there is SUGGESTIVE EVIDENCE that a careful, seasoned clinician observing a febrile infant for certain characteristics will have a greater "sensitivity" than will laboratory tests such as a white blood cell (WBC) count and ESR or C-reactive protein tests (4). The characteristics that indicate that an infant is at risk of the complications of bacteremia are shown in Table 1-1. The characteristics are drawn from a number of studies (4,6) that confirm the finding that careful observation and examination are more valid than laboratory tests. Repeated and detailed observation after appropriate antipyretic measures have been taken (45 to 60 minutes) is the major diagnostic approach.

Table 1-1. Clinical characteristics and the risk of complications of bacteremia

Clinical characteristic	Little risk	Moderate risk	Greater risk
Response to social overtures	Smiles repeatedly; if crying, stops in response to parental cuddling	Brief smile or does not stop crying for more than a few seconds	Anxious or apathetic or continues to cry
Play activity	Normal spontaneous play, or plays interactively with parent	Brief interest, then apathy or refusal	Refusal to play
Level of consciousness	Normal	Lethargic	Delirium, stupor, coma
Temperature	38.4°C or less	38.5–40°C	< 37 or > 40°C
Quality of cry	Strong cry, normal tone	Whimpering, sobbing	Weak, or moaning, or high-pitched
Respiratory effort	No distress	Tachypnea, mild indrawing	Severe, labored; marked indrawing

Occult bacteremia has been reported in approximately 5% of infants with temperatures of 39.5°C or more. For infants with fevers this high (especially if there are no focal signs helping to identify a treatable cause), routine blood cultures have been recommended, since a small percentage of these infants will develop complications of bacteremia, such as meningitis or pneumonia (7).

There is NO CLEAR EVIDENCE that febrile infants, including those with temperature of 39.5°C or more, are better off if blood cultures are performed than if they are not. It is probably more important to maintain close contact with the parents and to reexamine the infant, daily if necessary, than to routinely do blood cultures.

Children 2 years of age or older

Children 2 years old or older are at less risk of occult, life-threatening infection. Most infections causing fever in this age group are viral and self-limited. Otitis media and group A beta-hemolytic streptococcal infections are the most common treatable bacterial infections. If no focus of infection is found and the child does not appear toxic after appropriate antipyretic measures have been taken, the risk of missing occult, life-threatening bacterial infection is very remote and few, if any, laboratory tests should be done. If fever persists for more than 48 hours and no signs of symptoms such as cough, rhinitis, or diarrhea develop, then another physical examination is indicated. If there are still no findings, the approach should be based on how the child looks and whether the temperature is beginning to subside. If a fever of

38.5°C or more persists for more than 2 or 3 days, without focal signs, then CBC, ESR, urinalysis, and urine culture may be indicated; if there is cough or tachypnea, a chest radiograph should also be taken since occult bacterial pneumonia may be difficult to diagnose clinically.

MANAGEMENT

There are two aspects of the treatment of fever in infants and children: first, the treatment of the cause or presumed cause of the fever, and second, nonspecific antipyretic measures.

The specific treatments of the known causes—e.g., otitis media, pneumonia, urinary tract infections—are described in the relevant chapters in this section. A major issue is whether to give antibiotics to infants 3 to 24 months old who have rectal temperatures of more than 38.5°C but who have no focal cause in the attempt to prevent complications of occult bacteremia. There is SUGGESTIVE EVIDENCE of decreased bacterial complications in a group of infants with temperatures greater than 39.4°C who had elevated WBC and ESR and who were treated with intramuscular penicillin (7). This study has been attacked as having serious methodological problems, the most serious of which was grouping otitis media with meningitis to show a statistically significant difference in complications between the treated and untreated groups. If otitis media is removed as a "complication of bacteremia," the difference in serious bacterial complications between the two groups is not statistically significant (8). Another study (FIRM EVIDENCE) showed no difference between a group of febrile infants treated "expectantly" with antibiotics and a control group given placebo (9). Thus, infants more than 3 months old in whom there is no clear focus of infection should not routinely be treated with antibiotics.

Nonspecific antipyretic measures include physical and pharmacologic techniques. First, it should be established that lowering the fever is worthwhile. Arguments against treating fever are based on experimental studies that show that leukocyte motility, lymphocyte transformation, and interferon production are enhanced by fever. In addition, physical means of lowering temperature (sponging) are unpleasant, and pharmacologic agents (acetylsalicylic acid, acetaminophen) may have toxic effects. The arguments in favor of treating fever are twofold: first, there has never been a controlled clinical trial demonstrating that the treatment of fever prolongs or worsens illness, and second, fever not only makes people feel ill but it may cause them to look ill enough to motivate physicians to perform unnecessary and potentially dangerous tests, e.g., lumbar punctures, in an attempt to find a cause for the toxic appearance. The appropriate diagnostic and therapeutic approach to the infant or child with high fever of no apparent cause is contingent upon the child's appearance after appropriate antipyretic measures have been taken.

Tepid water is best for sponging the patient. Cold or cool water causes blood vessels in the skin to constrict, thereby preventing the heat from reaching the skin. The skin should not be dried with a towel, since it is the evaporation of water from the skin that causes heat to be released through it. Rubbing alcohol should not be used since it can be absorbed into the body. There is SUGGESTIVE EVIDENCE that sponging is not effective in lowering body temperature (10).

Pharmacologic agents such as acetaminophen or acetylsalicylic acid in doses of 10 mg/kg/ no more frequently than every 4 hours are effective. The maximum single dose for a 60-kg adolescent is 600 mg. Because there is SUGGESTIVE EVIDENCE of a relationship between infections with varicella and influenza and the development of Reye's syndrome in children given acetylsalicylic acid, acetaminophen is recommended for children whose fevers are suspected of being caused by either of these infections (11).

REFERENCES

1. De Angelis, C., Joffe, A., Willis, E., Wilson, M. Hospitalization v. outpatient treatment of young febrile infants. *Am. J. Dis. Child.* 137:1150–1152, 1983.
2. Greene, J.W., Hara, C., O'Connor, S., Altemeir, W.A. Management of febrile outpatient neonates. *Clin. Pediatr.* 20:375–380, 1981.
3. De Angelis, C., Joffe, A., Wilson, M., Willis, E. Iatrogenic risks and financial costs of hospitalizing febrile infants. *Am. J. Dis. Child.* 137:1146–1149, 1983.
4. Waskerwitz, S., Berkelhamer, J. Outpatient bacteremia: Clinical findings in children under two years with initial temperatures of 39.5 C or higher. *J. Pediatr.* 99:231–233, 1981.
5. McCarthy, P., Jekel, J., Dolan, T. Comparison of acute-phase reactants in pediatric patients with fever. *Pediatrics* 62:716–720, 1978.
6. Nelson, K.G. An index of severity for acute pediatric illness. *Am. J. Public Health* 70:804–807, 1980.
7. Carroll, W.L., Farrell, M.K., Singer, J.I., Jackson, M.A., Nobel, J.S., Lewis, E.D. Treatment of occult bacteremia: A prospective randomized clinical trial. *Pediatrics* 72:608–612, 1983.
8. Feldman, W. Treatment of occult bacteremia (Letter). *Pediatrics* 74:1131–1132, 1984.
9. Jaffe, D., Fleisher, G., Henretig, F. The effect of oral antibiotic therapy on febrile children with bacteremia: Preliminary report of a randomized trial (Abstract). *Am. J. Dis. Child.* 137:533, 1983.
10. Newman, J. Evaluation of sponging to reduce body temperature. *Can. Med. Assoc. J.* 132:641–642, 1985.
11. Reye Syndrome—United States, 1984. *M.M.W.R. Surveill. Summ.* 34:13–16, 1985.

2

UPPER RESPIRATORY PROBLEMS

RHINITIS

Prevalence

Rhinitis and pharyngitis are the illnesses that children most commonly develop. Infants do not usually develop upper respiratory tract infections (URI) until they are 3 to 4 months old; their maternal antibodies provide protection. Often, sneezing or evidence of nasal obstruction in an infant is interpreted as a URI. After the age of 4 months, URI begin to occur on the average of at least twice annually. When a child is exposed to many other children, such as in school or in a day-care center, the frequency of URI may rise to five or six times annually. Such infections may include rhinitis, pharyngitis, laryngitis, and, less commonly, sinusitis, alone or in combination with another infection.

Narrowing down

The most common causes of rhinitis are the 200 or more viral agents that have been identified over the past 20 years. Because of the prevalence of URI, the natural history of a viral URI is important, since deviation from the expected natural history is suggestive of another etiology for the symptoms (Fig. 2-1).

The URI caused by a virus is characterized initially by almost complete nasal obstruction accompanied by a low-grade fever (up to 38.5°C), sometimes headache and general malaise. There is a minimal amount of clear nasal discharge for approximately 24 hours. During the following 3 to 5 days a copious mucopurulent nasal discharge congests the nasal passages. Subsequently a yellowish mucopurulent discharge occurs for 2 to 3 days and then dries up. The normal course of the viral URI is completed in about 10 to 12 days. Development of a high fever early on, between days 1 and 4, in a suspected viral URI is suggestive of bacterial etiology. Prolongation of the natural history suggests either an allergy or a superimposed bacterial infection. In children, the mucopurulent discharge that starts between days 3 and 4 and

9

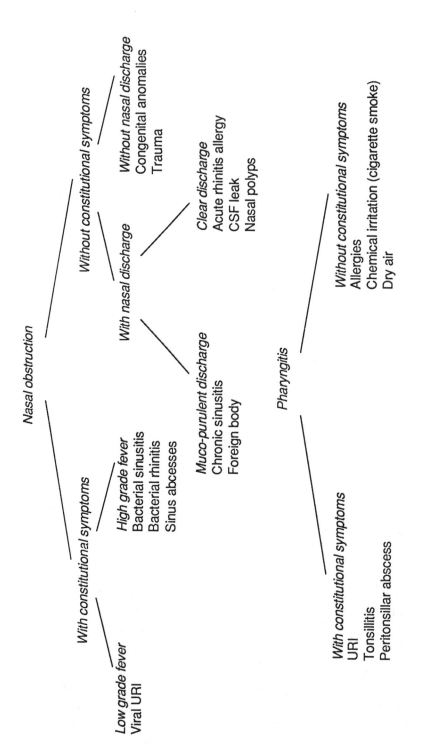

Figure 2-1. Narrowing down the problems of nasal obstruction and pharyngitis.

continues until day 10 is often irritating to the nares and to the upper lip. Coughing and other respiratory complaints may be secondary to a postnasal drip of mucopurulent discharge. Bacterial rhinitis is the most common cause of acute suppurative rhinitis or sinusitis. The organisms most commonly causing bacterial rhinitis include *Steptococcus pneumoniae*, other streptococci, *Haemophilus influenzae*, and, occasionally, *Staphylococcus aureus*.

Sinusitis is very rare in preschool-aged children, since children are born with only the ethmoid and maxillary sinuses open. Paranasal sinuses become clinically significant at about age 6 and the frontal sinuses between the ages of 8 and 10. Bacterial sinusitis is characterized by acute pain and a high fever, with copious mucopurulent discharge. Bacterial sinusitis in young children, although rare, is significant because of the risk of abscess formation and development of erosion through the ethmoid bones, causing osteomyelitis, and possibly meningitis and orbital cellulitis. Sinus abscesses are rare and usually occur after bacterial sinusitis. Rarely, they may lead to meningitis.

A lack of constitutional symptoms when a mucopurulent discharge is present in children over the age of 7 suggests chronic sinusitis, which is rare but usually bacterial in origin. The sinus is inflamed or infected on a chronic basis and polyps may be present. Radiographs may be of assistance in narrowing the diagnosis.

A mucopurulent discharge without constitutional symptoms in a child under the age of 6 suggests a foreign body. A foreign body in the nares produces an acute reaction, resulting in copious, foul-smelling discharge until the object is removed. The most useful diagnostic point is the history of a more acute onset than occurs in chronic sinusitis.

Allergic rhinitis is the most common cause of a clear nasal discharge over a period of weeks or months. Using the natural history of a viral URI as the baseline, frequent recurrences of clear discharge suggest allergic rhinitis. A family history of allergies and the presence of pets in the household may be discovered. If a nasal swab for cells is taken from a child with chronic allergic rhinitis, there will be a high percentage of eosinophils in the mucus. A blood count may show an elevated number of eosinophils. There is NO CLEAR EVIDENCE that children with chronic allergic rhinitis are more prone to viral and bacterial infections than those who do not have the problem (1). The appearance of the nasal mucosa, which is often described as boggy, with purplish discoloration and marked edema usually partially obstructing the nasal passages, helps confirm the diagnosis. Other distinguishing signs of allergic rhinitis include the so-called allergic salute, in which the child compresses the nares upward. There may be dark rings under both eyes. Allergic rhinitis may be characterized by mouth breathing and the oral shape characteristic of mouth breathing, with protrusion of the front teeth. There is NO CLEAR EVIDENCE demonstrating whether mouth breathing is secondary to the shape of the face and mouth, or whether chronic nasal obstruction causes the facial characteristics (2).

Nasal polyps may or may not cause a chronic clear discharge, but they often obstruct the nasal passages. Polyps can be seen on examination of the nasal chambers. Their surface is much paler than that of the normal mucosa. Polyps almost always accompany chronic allergic rhinitis, but cystic fibrosis must also be considered.

Cerebrospinal fluid rhinorrhea, a rare problem in children, usually follows a basal skull fracture. The clear rhinorrhea is usually aggravated by leaning forward. It is differentiated from a mucous discharge by testing the sugar content using a glucose dip stick. The presence of glucose confirms the presence of cerebrospinal fluid since there is no glucose in normal nasal mucus. Cerebrospinal fluid rhinorrhea is important because patients are at risk of bacterial invasion of the brain and meninges.

Nasal obstruction may be caused by congenital anomalies, such as choanal atresia, which is apparent almost immediately after birth because of breathing and feeding difficulties. Trauma may cause hematomas of the medial septum, with accompanying edema and obstruction.

Management

Although there are many treatments of viral URI available, both with and without prescription, clinical trials have shown NO CLEAR EVIDENCE that any intervention alters the natural history of the illness. Symptomatic management to overcome nasal obstruction and reduce discharge using decongestants may relieve discomfort but does not alter the natural history. The treatment of fever was discussed in Chapter 1. Nasal obstruction in young infants that causes feeding problems may be aided by the administration of normal saline drops.

Bacterial sinusitis must be treated vigorously with antibiotics, such as amoxicillin at a dosage of 40 mg/kg/24 hours in three divided doses or trimethoprim-sulfamethoxazole at 6 to 8 mg/kg/24 hours in two divided doses. Chronic sinusitis in adolescents may require draining the sinuses, although the use of both topical and systemic decongestants and antibiotics should be attempted before surgical intervention. Allergic rhinitis may be aided by environmental control for allergens, oral antihistamines, or topical sodium cromoglycate. Betamethasone may also be used topically. Foreign bodies are often removed in a simple office procedure: occasionally surgical intervention is required. CSF rhinorrhea requires neurosurgical management by an appropriate consultant. Nasal polyps also require surgery.

PHARYNGITIS

Prevalence

The prevalence of viral pharyngitis follows a pattern similar to that of viral URI. Tonsillitis is less frequent.

Narrowing down

Viral pharyngitis is usually accompanied by other symptoms of URI, including low-grade fever and nasal discharge (see Fig. 2-1). Viral infections of the pharynx usually produce erythema, with occasional edematous lymph nodes, but rarely is the pharynx covered with exudates. Lymphadenopathy in the submandibular region and along the sternomastoid muscles may be present, but the nodes are usually small and only slightly tender. The constitutional symptoms that usually accompany viral pharyngitis are relatively mild, compared with those of streptococcal pharyngitis.

Streptococcal pharyngitis includes marked tonsillar pharyngeal erythema and edema, marked anterior cervical lymphadenopathy, often with moderate to marked tonsillar pharyngeal exudates. Palatine stippling and erythema are often present. There is FIRM EVIDENCE that marked erythema of the pharynx and enlarged, tender lymph nodes in the neck have an 85% positive predictive value for streptococcal infection. The addition of palatine stippling and erythema of the soft palate has raised the positive predictive value to 89% (3). When these three signs are present, it has been argued that throat cultures are not necessary. Cultures should be taken in patients having only one of the above four signs, as it is much more difficult to differentiate bacterial infection from viral disease in them (4). The recent development and testing of in-office latex agglutination methods for determining the presence of streptococci improves the physician's ability to be more precise in differentiating viral from streptococcal pharyngitis. Recent studies have found a 92% positive predictive value for latex agglutination tests done in a clinic or office setting (5). Performing throat cultures on all children with pharyngitis is not desirable, as cultures will detect incidental carriers of streptococcal disease who may then be treated unnecessarily. Children less than 2 years old who have pharyngitis, are mildly febrile, and have no exudates should not be treated. Children who have the characteristics of a streptococcal throat accompanied by a high fever should be treated without a culture being taken. There is also debate as to whether follow-up cultures are necessary. Although there is NO CLEAR EVIDENCE, because of the extremely low incidence of rheumatic fever, follow-up cultures are probably not necessary unless the child develops a sore throat shortly after treatment.

Children, but more commonly adolescents, who present with a history of fatigue, fever, general malaise, a very inflamed pharynx with extensive exudates, and marked lymphadenopathy should be suspected of having infectious mononucleosis. Such a condition simulates severe streptococcal pharyngitis, but usually the onset occurs over a period of more than one week. The presence of other constitutional symptoms, such as splenomegaly, hepatomegaly, and extensive lymphadenopathy, may be helpful in narrowing the diagnosis. Frequently, children or adolescents presenting with these signs are administered penicillin or ampicillin; they subsequently develop a macular rash that is characteristic of infectious mononucleosis. A complete blood cell count, including a white cell count and a differential count, and a mono-spot test will differentiate infectious mononucleosis from those with streptococcal pharyngitis. Mononucleosis usually is characterized by marked lymphocytosis. Streptococcal pharyngitis usually causes an elevated white blood count with neutrophilia.

Recurrent tonsillitis often occurs in children in the 3- to 7-year age group because they are frequently exposed to other children and their immunity is relatively low. The rare child with large tonsils that interfere with swallowing, cause gagging, or interfere with breathing should be considered for tonsillectomy.

Allergic rhinitis and chronic sinusitis secondary to allergies in young children and adolescents may cause a postnasal drip and irritation of the posterior pharyngeal wall. This is usually accompanied by other symptoms of allergic rhinitis but not by constitutional symptoms. Investigation and treatment of the allergies may be indicated if symptomatic treatment is unsuccessful. Rarely is there more than minimal lymphadenopathy accompanying allergic inflammation of the pharynx.

In very cold climates where subzero temperatures frequently occur in winter, the air inside buildings becomes extremely dry. Without appropriate humidification of the environment, children may suffer from irritation of the posterior pharyngeal wall. This phenomenon is aggravated in mouth breathers. Children who are chronically exposed to sidestream smoke from cigarettes or to other chemical inhalants may suffer chronic posterior pharyngeal irritation with no infectious cause.

Management of pharyngitis

There is FIRM EVIDENCE that a 10-day course of penicillin is adequate for treatment of all streptococcal pharyngitis. Recurrent episodes of streptococcal pharyngitis should arouse the suspicion that the child is either exposed to a carrier or is not complying with the treatment regimen (3). With frequent recurrences, consideration should be given to a course of penicillin of more than 10 days.

Criteria commonly used in deciding whether tonsillectomy should be considered include seven episodes of tonsillitis within a 1-year period, five or more episodes in each of the 2 preceding years, or three or more episodes in each of the 3 preceding years. A randomized trial to test the benefit of tonsillectomy in children in whom these criteria were met yielded SUGGESTIVE EVIDENCE of no significant benefit in children undergoing tonsillectomy in comparison with children in the control group who did not undergo tonsillectomies. During the first 2 years after tonsillectomy, there were fewer throat infections, but by the third year after the operation the frequency of throat infections was equivalent to that in the control group. No major adverse effects were observed in either group during the trial. This trial suggests that there is little long-term benefit of tonsillectomy unless the airway or swallowing is impeded (6).

If there are no constitutional symptoms and if all the other possible causes of posterior pharyngeal irritation have been eliminated, the use of a children's vaporizer should reduce pharyngeal irritation. If it appears that pharyngeal irritation is secondary to exposure to side-stream smoke, this should be pointed out to smoking adults and attempts made to reduce the child's exposure.

REFERENCES

1. Tarlo, S., Broder, I., Spence, L. A prospective study of respiratory infection in adult asthmatics and their normal spouses. *Clin. Allergy* 9:293–301, 1979.
2. Sassoun, V., Shnorhokian, H., Berry, Q., et al. Influence of potential allergic rhinitis on facial type. *J. Allergy Clin. Immunol.* 69:149–155, 1982.
3. Brazie, D.B., Dennie, F.W., Dillon, H.C., Stillerman, N., Nelson, J.D., McCracken, G.H. Jr. Difficult management problems in children with streptococcal pharyngitis. *Pediatr. Infect. Dis.* 4:10–13, 1985.
4. Berkowitz, J. Culturing throat swabs. End of an era? *Pediatrics* 107:85, 1985.
5. Gerber, J. Latex agglutination to identify streptococcal antigen. *J. Pediatr.* 107:85–88, 1985.
6. Paradise, J.C., Bluestone, C.D., Bachman, R.N., Colborn, D.K., Bernard, B.S., Taylor, F.H., Rogers, K.D., Schwarzbach, R.H. Stool, S.E., Friday, G.A., Smith, I.H., Saez, C.A. Efficacy of tonsillectomy for recurrent throat infection in severely affected children. *N. Engl. J. Med.* 310:674–683, 1984.

3

EAR PROBLEMS

In children, the major complaints involving the ear are pain, short- or long-term hearing deficits, and discharge. Most of these problems are caused by ear infections; consequently, in this chapter we concentrate on otitis media and otitis externa. Hearing deficits not associated with infection are uncommon, but it is very important to diagnose them early in a child's life; thus the problem of deafness is discussed at length.

PREVALENCE

Ear pain due to otitis media is very common. More that two-thirds of children will have at least one attack in the first 3 years of life (1); thereafter the incidence declines. The reasons for the high prevalence of otitis media in infancy and the decline at 3 years are unknown.

Ear pain due to otitis externa is less common in infants and increases with age, presumably because older children swim more often. Exact prevalence data are not available.

Deafness in childhood is, fortunately, uncommon; severe bilateral congenital deafness is found in 1 in 2,000 newborns (2). Mild unilateral hearing problems (inability to hear at 25 decibels) in kindergarten students are much more common and are usually the result of fluid accumulation in the middle ear following otitis media. These problems are short-lived and occur in 7 to 30% of children, depending on the season and the prevalence of respiratory and middle ear infections. The high-prevalence months in northern climates are November through April (10).

The prevalence of discharge from the ear is unknown, but it has been reduced since the advent of the widespread, early use of antibiotics for the treatment of acute otitis media.

16

EAR PAIN

Narrowing down

The clues leading to the diagnosis of acute otitis media, otitis externa, and furuncles in the ear canal are shown in Table 3-1.

Diagnosis

Given a history of ear pain, or, in infants, of irritability and fever, the diagnosis is best made by otoscopic inspection. Although the child's crying may make the tympanic membrane slightly red, a unilaterally red tympanic membrane that is bulging indicates acute otitis media, which should be treated. Movement of the pinna is not painful in acute otitis media but is very painful in otitis externa or if there is a furuncle in the canal. Pneumatic otoscopy and tympanometry will show fluid in the middle ear but cannot distinguish pus from a sterile effusion. These procedures are not necessary in most clinical situations. Fever and a red, bulging tympanic membrane are virtually diagnostic of acute otitis media. However, in many cases fever may be mild or absent. If there is hyperemia and pain even without bulging, a bacterial infection may be present, which warrants treatment.

Tympanocentesis and culture of the middle-ear fluid are not necessary. The results of throat cultures do not correlate with those of middle-ear cultures and neither is indicated. Cultures of ear exudates usually reflect superinfection; the organisms identified are rarely causative. The white blood cell count (WBC) does not necessarily imply bacterial infection; that is, with a WBC in the "viral" range, bacteria may be isolated from the middle ear.

Management

There are two aspects to the treatment of ear pain: first, nonspecific treatment of the pain, and, second, specific treatment of the cause of the pain. For non-

Table 3-1. Narrowing down and diagnosis of ear pain

	History	Tympanic membrane	Canal
Acute otitis media	Younger children; acute onset, often fever	Red, bulging, rarely perforated	Not painful on movement of ear
Otitis externa	Swimming; may put bobby pins in canal seborrhea	If visible, normal	Canal swollen; pus; very tender when ear moved
Furuncle in canal	Older children; often acne or seborrhea	Normal	Furuncle visible in canal; very tender when ear moved

specific treatment of earache, analgesic drugs such as acetylsalicylic acid or acetominophen can be given in doses of 10 mg/kg, up to 300 milligrams every 4 to 6 hours as long as is necessary for pain relief. Children over 10 years of age may be administered up to two adult tablets of acetylsalicylic acid or acetominophen every 4 to 6 hours. It is rarely necessary to administer analgesics for more than 24 hours for ear pain. There is NO CLEAR EVI-DENCE that topical therapy (drops) eases the pain of otitis media.

Specific treatment

For *acute otitis media*, the mainstays of treatment are antibiotics. A recent study (3) suggested that the outcome in children given antibiotics was not much different from that in children given placebo. However, that study pro-vided NO CLEAR EVIDENCE, since it was methodologically flawed. Statisti-cal analysis of the data presented yielded conclusions quite different from those published by the investigators, namely, that the complication rate in treated children was strikingly lower than that in untreated children (4).

In areas where the resistance of *Haemophilus influenzae* to ampicillin is low, amoxicillin in a dose of 40 mg/kg/day in three divided doses is recommended as the drug of choice. To determine what the resistance rate of *H. influenzae* is in your community, contact the local microbiologist or laboratory that han-dles most of the bacterial cultures from children.

There is FIRM EVIDENCE that trimethoprim-sulfamethoxazole is a very good alternative and equal in cost. It can be administered at a dosage of 8 mg/ kg trimethoprim and 40 mg/kg sulfamethoxazole per 24 hours, in two divided doses (5). This antibiotic has the additional advantage of requiring only a twice-per-day administration, which enhances compliance. A course of anti-biotics is recommended for 10 days, although there is NO CLEAR EVI-DENCE that 10 days of therapy is more effective than 7 days or less effective than 14 days of therapy.

Oral cefaclor is quite effective in the treatment of acute otitis media but is more expensive than the afore-mentioned antibiotics.

Erythromycin-sulfonamide combinations are also effective and reason-able in cost, and are an excellent alternative for penicillin-sensitive children. For children more than 8 years old, an age group in which *H. influenzae* is an unusual cause of acute otitis media, penicillin V, 250 mg four times a day, can be prescribed. For older children who are allergic to penicillin, erythromycin, 30 mg/kg/24 hours, is effective. New antibiotics, such as ampicillins with added clavulanic acid to overcome resistant *H. influenzae* (Augmentin, Clavu-lan) are expensive. There is NO CLEAR EVIDENCE that they are superior to the antibiotics currently used.

Antihistamines (6) and decongestants (7) have been shown to be ineffec-tive (FIRM EVIDENCE) in the treatment of acute otitis media.

Myringotomy or tympanocentesis are rarely indicated in cases of acute otitis media. If a child's fever or pain do not respond to treatment in 48 to 72 hours, he or she should be reexamined. If there is no improvement in the appearance of the tympanic membrane, the causative organism (most likely *H. influenzae*) is probably resistant to ampicillin. Trimethoprim-sulfamethoxazole, cefaclor, or erythromycin-sulfonamide should be effective.

Some preschool-aged children are otitis-prone, that is, they have three or more attacks of acute otitis media in one 6-month period. For *recurrent acute otitis media*, there is FIRM EVIDENCE that long-term (3 to 6 months, or more if necessary) prophylactic administration of antimicrobial drugs successfully reduces the number of attacks. This form of therapy (e.g., 75 mg/kg/day sulfonamide in two divided doses for 3 months) is inexpensive and efficacious in families that comply with the regimen (8). There is FIRM EVIDENCE that adenoidectomy is not effective in reducing recurrent attacks of acute otitis media (9).

The role of recurrent acute otitis media in the pathogenesis of speech and learning problems has not been established.

In children at risk of otitis externa (swimmers, children with eczema or seborrhea, habitual ear-canal scratchers) the presence of *discharge*, with pain on movement of the external ear, merits topical therapy. Swimming should be temporarily discontinued. The canal should be gently cleaned using a cotton swab (if tolerated) or gently syringed before ear drops containing antibiotics with hydrocortisone are applied. Combinations of neomycin and bacitracin or polymyxin with hydrocortisone, or an otic solution of chloramphenicol with hydrocortisone may be used, four drops in the canal four times a day. Topical gentamicin is also effective.

Rarely, the skin around the ear will be red, which suggests cellulitis. Oral cloxacillin and amoxicillin, each at 50 to 100 mg/kg/24 hours every 6 hours, can be prescribed at first; if there is no improvement in 24 to 48 hours, intravenous antibiotics may be required. It may be necessary to use intravenous chloramphenicol if resistant *H. influenzae* are suspected.

For a *furuncle in the ear canal*, warm water should be applied in the canal four or five times a day to shorten the course of the boil. Antibiotics or surgical drainage (by an ear, nose, and throat surgeon) may be indicated.

HEARING PROBLEMS

Narrowing down

Congenital deafness may be inherited in an autosomal dominant or recessive pattern. A family history of deafness should prompt careful monitoring of an infant's hearing by both parents and doctor. Intrauterine infections such as rubella and the administration of ototoxic drugs (e.g., aminoglycosides) to the mother during pregnancy may produce deafness in her child. Perinatal factors, such as severe hyperbilirubinemia, administration of ototoxic drugs to the newborn, or meningitis, also put the infant at risk. With new audiometric technology of brainstem evoked potentials, no infant is too young to be tested for deafness.

In infants who are at little risk of congenital deafness, the best screening is provided by the parents (see Chapter 14). There generally is, unfortunately, a long delay (1 year) between the parents' suspecting deafness in their child and the physician's initiation of appropriate management. There is FIRM EVIDENCE that early detection makes a significant difference in the course of the disorder (2). By 3 months of age infants should look in the direction of the speaker; even earlier, they should demonstrate a startle response to loud noises. Infants who do not respond in this manner may be deaf, mentally retarded, or autistic. Older infants and children who experience a significant delay in language acquisition but who are otherwise socially responsive and developmentally normal are most likely hard of hearing.

Helpful clues for diagnosing the cause of a hearing problem are shown in Table 3-2.

Management

The infant who is suspected of having a hearing problem or who is at high risk of deafness should undergo a thorough audiologic assessment as soon as possible. If deafness is confirmed, management by a team consisting of an audiologist, a developmental pediatrician, an otolaryngologist, and a speech therapist, is indicated. The infant will be fitted with hearing aids and monitored by experts in speech and hearing for many years.

The primary care physician's role is to coordinate the total care of the child and to be supportive of the family. Since several specialists are usually involved managing the child's hearing problem, the child's and the family's other health care needs may be neglected. The physician should be aware that many families have great difficulty coping with their grief for and guilt about a deaf child (see Chapter 26).

The usual causes of hearing problems in preschool-aged and school-aged children are serous otitis media and recurrent acute otitis media. For the medical management of these problems, see the section in this chapter on the treatment of recurrent acute otitis media. In addition to medical management, surgical therapy is often used. The insertion of ventilation tubes may dramatically improve hearing in the short term, but spontaneous improvement of hearing within 3 months in non-operated ears is equivalent to the improvement in ears with ventilation tubes (11). In addition, complications secondary to the surgical insertion of tubes are not rare.

In children who have fluid in the middle ear confirmed by tympanometry, tympanocentesis may reveal bacteria in the middle-ear fluid in the absence of fever, pain, or redness of the tympanic membrane. If hearing loss is proven, a 3- to 6-month course of prophylactic antimicrobial therapy should be given. There is FIRM EVIDENCE that medical treatment usually results in improved hearing (8). If, after 3 to 6 months of medical management, there is no im-

Table 3-2. Narrowing down and diagnosis of hearing problems

	Infants	Preschool-aged	School-aged
History	Intrauterine infection, severe jaundice, maternal ototoxic drugs, meningitis, family history of deafness	Family history of deafness; meningitis; delay or absence of speech; abnormal response to verbal requests; history of recurrent otitis	Inattentiveness in class; turns television volume up; has to look at speaker to understand speech
Physical examination	Not responsive to spoken sounds by 3 months; no startle response to loud noises by 3 months; other stigmata of rubella syndrome	Serous or recurrent acute otitis media fluid in middle ear; dullness and loss of light reflex of tympanic membrane; no evidence of autism or global delay	As in preschool-aged children
Laboratory tests	Auditory brainstem evoked potentials	Tympanometry: mature 4-year-old may respond to pure-tone audiogram; other specialized tests by experienced audiologists as necessary	Pure-tone audiogram; tympanometry

provement in pure-tone and tympanometric audiometry, the child should be referred to an otolaryngologist for possible insertion of ventilation tubes.

EAR DISCHARGE

Narrowing down and diagnosis

It is sometimes difficult to tell whether pus in the ear canal is coming from a perforated tympanic membrane or is being produced in the canal itself. The removal of the pus using a cotton swab can be gently attempted but should be discontinued if it produces too much discomfort. If the tympanic membrane can be visualized and a perforation seen, the diagnosis is otitis media. If not, and movement of the pinna causes considerable pain, the most likely diagnosis is otitis externa, especially in swimmers. Blood coming from the ear canal (in a child who has not scratched the canal) may be the result of head trauma and a basal skull fracture. Chronically draining ears are rare in children who have access to good medical care; nevertheless, in native American children, chronic drainage due to chronic otitis media with perforation of the tympanic membrane is still prevalent. A rare cause of chronically draining ears is histiocytosis X; children with this condition are chronically ill, fail to thrive, and have distinctive lesions of the skin, bone, and viscera.

Laboratory tests are of little assistance in diagnosing the average case of acute discharge. The correlation between the organisms cultured from the canal and those that cause the infection is usually poor. Since the organisms in the canal are usually secondary invaders, canal cultures are not helpful in diagnosis and management.

Management

Analgesics and antibiotics should be administered as for acute otitis media if the discharge is due to the perforation of the tympanic membrane that occasionally develops in that condition. If the discharge is due to otitis externa, topical therapy is indicated.

REFERENCES

1. Bluestone, C.D. Otitis media in children: To treat or not to treat. *N. Engl. J. Med.* 306:1399–1404, 1982.
2. Northern, J.L., Downs, M.P. *Hearing in children.* Baltimore: Williams and Wilkins, 1974, p. 97.
3. Van Buchem, F.L., Dunk, J.H.M., Van't Hof., H.M.A. Therapy of acute otitis media: Myringotomy, antibiotics or neither? *Lancet* 2:883–887, 1981.
4. Feldman, W. Management of acute otitis media. *Lancet* 1:111, 1982.
5. Feldman, W., Richardson, H., Rennie, B., Dawson, P. A trial comparing cefaclor with co-trimoxazole in the treatment of acute otitis media. *Arch. Dis. Child.* 57:594–597, 1982.
6. O'Shea, J.S., Langenbrunner, D.J., McCloskey, D.E., Pezzullo, J.C., Regan, J.B. Childhood serious otitis media. *Clin. Pediatr.* 21:150–153, 1982.
7. Olson, A.L., Klein, S.W., Charney, E., MacWhinney, B., McInerny, T.K., Miller, R.L., Nazarian, L.F., Cunninghan, D. Prevention and therapy of serious otitis media by oral decongestant: A double-blind study in pediatric practice. *Pediatrics* 61:679–684, 1978.
8. Liston, T.E., Foshee, W.S., Pierson, W.D. Sulfisoxazole chemoprophylaxis for frequent otitis media. *Pediatrics* 71:524–530, 1983.
9. Bluestone, C.D. Personal communication. 1982.
10. Feldman, W., Sackett, B., Milner, R.A., Gilbert, S. Effects of preschool screening for vision and hearing on prevalence of vision and hearing problems 6-12 months later. *Lancet* 2:1014–1016, 1980.
11. Brown, M.J.K.M., Richards, S.H., Ambeguokar, A.G. Grommets and the glue ear: A five year follow-up of a controlled trial. *J. R. Soc. Med.* 71:353–356, 1978.

4
VOMITING AND REGURGITATION

PREVALENCE

Vomiting is an extremely common problem in children; almost no child goes through the first 10 years of life without suffering several episodes of vomiting. Although vomiting is most commonly a symptom of a viral infection, most systemic illnesses that afflict a child can stimulate vomiting. In infants less than one year old, it is important to differentiate pathologic vomiting from regurgitation or chalasia. Approximately 40% of infants regurgitate some stomach contents. If the infant's stomach is full, he may regurgitate, but usually no more than 20% of the food consumed at any feeding.

NARROWING DOWN

An infant is usually not distressed by regurgitation, which generally occurs within less than one hour of a feeding. Weight loss may be associated with significant vomiting but rarely with regurgitation. Narrowing down the cause of vomiting is aided by an understanding of the pathophysiology and thus the source of the stimulation of the reflex reaction (Fig. 4-1). The stimulus to vomit can originate in the stomach, duodenum and intestinal tract, the vomiting center in the brain, the vestibular apparatus, or the visual, auditory, or olfactory systems (1). The history and physical examination are of major importance in determining which of the possible sources of activation of the vomiting reflex is most likely.

Mechanical causes of vomiting in the stomach or intestine

Infants from birth to 3 months vomit because of either stimulus by toxins from a variety of pathogens or mechanical obstruction secondary to pyloric stenosis. Pyloric stenosis occurs most commonly in firstborn males, in whom the incidence is as high as 1 in 200 (see Table 15-1 in Chapter 15). It is characterized by vomiting within 1 to 2 hours of feeding and classically involves projectile vomiting, although this usually occurs only when the obstruction is almost complete (2). As the obstruction increases there is some evidence of abdominal distention; very large quantities of stomach contents and liquids accumulate and ultimately are lost. Pyloric stenosis should be suspected in any child between 2 weeks and 3 months of age who experiences increasingly frequent and copious vomiting episodes accompanied by either loss of weight or no weight gain. A high level of suspicion and early detection will prevent severe malnutrition and life-threatening electrolyte imbalance. Other processes that cause mechanical obstruction of the intestine can result in fecal vomiting (3). Conditions such as hepatitis or peritonitis may produce nausea and vomiting (4).

Infectious causes of vomiting

Infections that result in vomiting in children less than 3 months old should be assessed very carefully because of their rare, serious implications (see Chap-

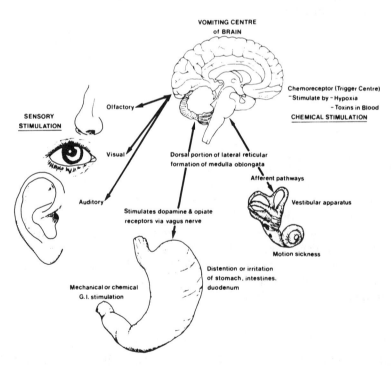

Figure 4-1. Physiology of mechanisms stimulating vomiting. (Courtesy of the Ottawa Civic Hospital.)

ter 1). Vomiting of acute onset after 3 months of age through the first year of life is usually caused by infection. Bacterial and viral toxins stimulate chemical sensors in the stomach, which stimulate the brain center that induces vomiting (5). Therefore, infections of the ears, throat, lung, and gastrointestinal or urinary tract must be ruled out in any child who is febrile and has a history of vomiting. Other mechanical causes of vomiting in young children include chemical irritation of sensors in the stomach by ingested aspirin, cough or cold remedies, alcohol, and a variety of drugs, all of which may irritate the stomach and duodenum. Children more than 1 year old with recurrent vomiting may rarely have a duodenal ulcer.

Brainstem causes of vomiting

Brain injury or other conditions that increase intracranial pressure by compressing the brainstem area may produce vomiting. Vomiting during or after anesthesia is likely due to chemical stimulation. Childhood migraine often causes vomiting and is associated with headaches, a positive family history for migraine, and complete absence of neurological findings. A condition called cyclic vomiting is occasionally seen in children between the ages of 3 and 10, in whom episodes of severe and sometimes protracted vomiting lasting for 2 to 3 days occur three or four times a year (6). This might be caused by a migraine-like ischemia of the brainstem. Chemicals may directly stimulate the vomiting center of the brain. Anticancer drugs are the most common cause of this type of vomiting. Endocrine disorders such as diabetic ketoacidosis and hypercalcemia secondary to hyperparathyrodism may induce vomiting. Uremia or marked electrolyte imbalance may also precipitate central-nervous-system vomiting. Vomiting because of salicylate intoxication may be caused by stomach irritation as well as central-nervous-system effects of acidosis.

In children with Reye's syndrome, vomiting may be due to cerebral edema or liver involvement. Vomiting because of motion sickness is more common in young children than in adults. The reasons for the increased sensitivity of the semicircular canals in children remain unclear. Inflammation, infection, or trauma to the semicircular canals or increased pressure in the middle ear may induce vomiting. A vomiting response that originates in the semicircular canals is often accompanied by vertigo and nystagmus, tinnitus, or hearing changes, all of which help clarify the diagnosis.

Psychological causes of vomiting

Visual, emotional, and other stimuli may induce vomiting. Severe forms of psychologically induced vomiting, such as anorexia nervosa and bulimia, are relatively rare in young children but do occur in adolescents; they are reviewed elsewhere (Chapter 17). Certain smells, sights, or even the appearance of some foods may induce recurrent vomiting in young children. Children become conditioned to develop nausea and vomiting under specific circumstances. For example, children receiving chemotherapy may vomit when they enter the treatment building, before they receive any drugs.

DIAGNOSIS

Pyloric stenosis is usually confirmed by abdominal ultrasound or barium swallow. Chalasia is usually a clinical diagnosis in the thriving infant who regurgitates frequently but not enough quantity to interfere with normal growth. Fever and other signs of infection—ear pain, dysuria, diarrhea—are almost always associated with infectious causes of vomiting. Chemical causes are usually clear from the history, but the determination of blood salicylate levels may be necessary to confirm acetylsalicylic acid intoxication. Trauma or other conditions causing raised intracranial pressure are usually evident from the history. A full or bulging fontanelle in an infant or papilledema in an older child along with headaches, changes in personality, and/or an altered level of consciousness confirm the diagnosis. A computerized tomographic scan may be necessary to demonstrate the cause of raised intracranial pressure, but this test is usually ordered by a specialist.

Reye's syndrome should be suspected in a child who has had a recent infection and develops vomiting, hyperventilation, and changes in personality and sensorium. Blood ammonia levels will be elevated, as will be liver enzyme levels. Other causes of vomiting are almost always evident in the history, for example, polyuria and polydipsia in diabetic ketoacidosis. Blood glucose levels, electrolyte levels, and acid-base levels confirm that diagnosis.

MANAGEMENT

Careful history-taking and physical examination will usually point to the probable primary cause of vomiting. Psychological causes may be more difficult to detect but should be suspected when more common causes are unlikely and when the vomiting appears to be stress-related. The management of nausea and vomiting is principally the management of the underlying condition.

Regurgitation is influenced by the position of the gastric air bubble in relation to the cardia. There is FIRM EVIDENCE that positioning a baby prone with the head elevated places the gastric air bubble directly below the cardia so that the gas expelled in a burp is not accompanied by food, thus reducing or eliminating regurgitation (7). Mechanical obstructions must be dealt with surgically. Inflammation or irritation of the gastrointestinal tract by infections or toxic causes is usually self-limited. Frequently, in small children, vomiting brought on by infectious diseases can be controlled by frequent intake of small quantities of clear fluids. If the stomach is acutely inflamed, large quantities of fluids may distend the stomach and stimulate the vomiting center. There is SUGGESTIVE EVIDENCE that measures such as sipping or swallowing tablespoons of fluids every 10 minutes is the most desirable approach (8); the fluid should be one containing some carbohydrate, such as fruit juice, a soft drink or sweetened tea, to replace the electrolytes lost in vomiting. A so-called BRAT diet can be added to the regimen once the clear fluids have been tolerated for 6 to 8 hours. The BRAT diet consists of bananas, rice, applesauce, and toast. Small, frequent feedings are preferable to a few larger ones. Bland foods may reduce further irritation of the gastrointestinal tract. The use of antacids may be helpful to reduce the effects of gastritis. Drugs that reduce the sensitivity of the vomiting center are controversial: Drug therapy consists of antihistamines such as diphenhydramine. There is FIRM EVIDENCE that diphenhydramine (5mg/kg/24 hours) may reduce the tendency to vomit but it causes drowsiness, which may mask other symptoms (9).

Vomiting that results in either dehydration or electrolyte imbalances may require the intravenous replacement of electrolytes and fluids for a period of 12 to 24 hours. Persistent vomiting in infants, in spite of their taking frequent small sips of clear fluids, and the early signs of dehydration are indications for hospital admission and intravenous therapy. This is particularly critical in young infants, who may rapidly become more than 5% dehydrated (see Chapter 27).

Vomiting secondary to motion sickness may be alleviated by the use of antihistamines before the start of the trip. The management of the psychological causes of vomiting ranges from removing specific factors that precipitate the vomiting to intensive behavioral therapy. The management of anorexia nervosa and bulimia is discussed in Chapter 17. The treatment of vomiting induced by migraine is dealt with in Chapter 22.

REFERENCES

1. Gershorn, M., Erde, S. The nervous system of the gut. *Gastroenterology.* 80:1571–1594, 1981.
2. Barison, H.L., Wang, S.C. Physiology and pharmacology of vomiting. *Pharmacol. Rev.* 5:193–230, 1953.
3. Sharma, R.N., Dubey, P.C., Dixit, K.C., Bhargava, K.P. Neural pathways of emesis associated with experimental intestinal obstruction in dogs. *Indian J. Med. Res.* 60:291–295, 1972.
4. Walton, F.E., Moore, R.M., Graham, E.A. The nerve pathways in the vomiting of periotonitis. *Surgery* 22:829–837, 1931.

5. Martin, W.J., Marcus, S. Relation of pyrogenic and emetic properties of enterobacterial endotoxin and of staphylococcal enterotoxin. *J. Bacteriol.* 87:1019–1026, 1964.
6. Hout, C.S., Stickler, G.B. A study of 44 children with the syndrome of recurrent (cyclic) vomiting. *Pediatrics* 22:775–780, 1960.
7. Myers, W.F., Herbst, J.J. Effectiveness of positioning therapy for gastroesophageal reflex. *Pediatrics* 69:768–772, 1982.
8. Santosham, N., Burns, B., et al. Oral rehydration therapy for acute diarrhea in ambulatory children in the United States. *Pediatrics* 76:159–166, 1985.
9. Gellis, S., Kagan, B. *Management of Vomiting—Current Pediatric Therapy,* vol. 10. Philadelphia: W.B. Saunders, 1982, p. 169.

5

BOWEL PROBLEMS

Some of the more common problems of the gastrointestinal tract that occur in children are described in other chapters (see Chapter 4 and Chapter 22 for vomiting and recurrent abdominal pain, respectively). In this chapter several common problems are dealt with in detail: diarrhea, constipation, and acute abdominal pain. Less common problems such as blood in the stool and fecal incontinence are also discussed.

PREVALENCE

The exact prevalences of diarrhea, constipation, acute abdominal pain, blood in the stool, and fecal soiling are unknown, largely because the definitions of these problems are vague. In addition, parents react to these problems differently; some will not seek help for their child's severe diarrhea until there is dehydration while others will consult a physician if their perfectly healthy infant has a single loose stool. Although hospitalization rates for these illnesses represent only the tip of the iceberg, they are shown in Table 5-1. Of all these conditions, acute diarrhea is the most common, especially in infants; it accounts for approximately 16% of all hospital admissions of children 1 year old or younger (1).

ACUTE DIARRHEA

Narrowing down

Acute diarrhea is defined as the passage of stools containing more water and electrolytes than is normal over a period of a week or less. Acute diarrhea is most serious in infants, because the loss of fluid relative to their weight and surface area can be great. In addition, they cannot communicate that they are

Table 5-1. Hospitalization rates for children with bowel problems, 1979–84

Condition	Mean annual number of children admitted
Diarrhea	720
Acute appendicitis	199
Gastrointestinal bleeding, including inflammatory bowel disease	30

Children's Hospital of Eastern Ontario, 1979–1984.

dehydrated by complaining of thirst. Frequent changes of an infant's diapers because of watery diarrhea may result in decreased urine volume's going unnoticed.

The most common cause of acute diarrhea in babies is gastrointestinal infection. Most cases are caused by viruses, especially rotavirus.

Mothers breast-feeding their infants often complain that the infants have frequent, loose stools. In thriving breast-fed infants, as many as six to twelve stools every 24 hours, even if green in color, may be entirely normal (2). Some breast-fed infants with allergies to cow's milk may develop diarrhea or colic when their mothers drink cow's milk. Infants given antibiotics for infection elsewhere, for example, otitis media, may develop frequent, loose stools.

Diagnosis

The diagnosis of acute diarrhea is usually made by the parents, who notice that their child passes atypically watery stools. The important clinical aspects relate to evidence of dehydration, that is, has the infant lost more fluids and electrolytes than the parents have been able to replace? The clinical features that indicate the degree of dehydration are shown in Table 5-2.

Acute infectious diarrhea, most often caused by rotavirus, is frequently associated with vomiting. In about 50% of infants with rotavirus gastroenteritis, there is also evidence of upper respiratory infection. Rotavirus is the major cause of diarrhea in infants during the winter in temperate climates. Bacteria cause fewer than 10% of cases of infantile diarrhea; children with bacterial diarrhea rarely require antimicrobial therapy, since most cases are self-limited. Stool cultures for *Salmonella, Shigella, Yersinia, Campylobacter,* or enterotoxic *Escherichia coli* are needed only for those infants whose diarrhea follows an atypical course, that is, high fever, bloody diarrhea, or prolonged symptoms, or if there is an outbreak of diarrhea in, for example, a school or day-care center.

Table 5-2. Signs of dehydration in children

	Mild	Moderate	Severe
Central nervous system status	Playful, smiling alert	Irritable but alert	Lethargic, coma
Anterior fontanelle	Normal	Slightly sunken	Very depressed
Eyes	Still tearing, eyes appear normal	Few tears, eyes appear sunken	No tears, eyes very sunken
Blood pressure, pulse, respirations	Slight tachycardia	Pulse rate high, blood pressure normal, respiratory rate slightly increased	Pulse rapid and thready, blood pressure low, rapid respiratory rate, shocky
Urine ouput	Slightly decreased	Still voiding, scant amounts	Oliguria or anuria
Skin turgor	Normal	Slight loss of elasticity	Marked loss of elasticity
Weight loss (if known)	Less than 5%	5–10%	10%

Breast-fed babies who have frequent, loose stools merely need to be weighed on several consecutive office visits to ensure continuing gain; once this is established the diagnosis of normal breast-milk stools is confirmed.

To diagnose an allergy to cow's milk, a relatively rare phenomenon, milk must be removed from the diet and replaced with a soybean-milk preparation. If the diarrhea disappears, then several weeks later another challenge with cow's milk is required. If diarrhea again occurs and is again alleviated by soybean milk, then the diagnosis is secure. Many infants with this problem outgrow it by the age of 2. The second challenge is necessary to prove that cow's milk formula is causally related to the diarrhea because the soybean substitutes are so much more expensive than cow's milk formula and some infants will require them for months to years. In addition, some infants with cow's milk allergy are also sensitive to soybean protein. Infants who react with diarrhea to both cow's milk and soy formula should be referred to a specialist skilled in dealing with these problems.

Antibiotic-induced diarrhea is relatively common with the administration of broad-spectrum antibiotics; the diarrhea usually clears up within a few days when the antibiotic is discontinued.

Management

Since gastroenteritis in most children has a viral cause, and since antibiotics usually are not indicated even in bacterial enteritis, the major emphasis in management is on the prevention and treatment of dehydration. For mildly dehydrated children it is essential to ensure adequate oral intake of fluids. In the developed world and in well-nourished children, there is FIRM EVIDENCE that commercially available solutions or powders containing glucose and electrolytes are no better than ½ strength apple juice, carbonated drinks, or ½ strength liquid, flavored gelatin (3).

The physician, having assessed by clinical examination (and weighing, if a recent, previous weight is known) that the child is less than 5% dehydrated, should calculate the basic fluid requirements using an empirical formula: 100 ml minus 3 multiplied by age (years) per kg per 24 hours. Then add 25 ml/kg/ 24 hours for mild dehydration. Thus, a 3-year-old weighing 15 kg should have 100 ml − (3 × 3) = 91 ml × 15 kg − 1,365 ml for maintenance fluid intake plus 25 ml × 15 kg = 375 ml to compensate for any deficit. The total is 1,740 milliliters, or, for simplicity, 1,800 milliliters of fluid in the next 24 hours, which is 1,800 divided by 24 hours or 75 milliliters per hour. A trial of one or two ounces in the office or in the patient's home (in the unlikely event of a house call) or as monitored by telephone (if the physician knows the family, the child is more than 6 months old, and the parents are reliable) is indicated to ensure that the child can keep the fluids down.

Infants less than 6 months old with acute diarrhea should be seen by the physician early on for an assessment of hydration. These younger infants are particularly prone to significant, rapid volume depletion and must be monitored carefully. In the event of vomiting shortly after ingesting fluid the child should be assessed for hydration. Another trial of fluids by mouth is indicated. In one recent study, the authors found very few infants with mild gastroenteritis who could not be rehydrated orally (3).

In the example given above, the parents should be instructed to administer 75 milliliters (2.5 ounces) by mouth every hour for the next 4 to 6 hours, and to report to the physician how the child is doing at that time. If there is vomiting, it may be better to give 1 ounce every 20 minutes. In infants, if the degree of dehydration is not clear, or if the reliability of the parents is not known, it is better to admit the child to the hospital for observation. After admission, a further trial of fluids by mouth is indicated unless the child vomits persistently or there are continuous fecal losses that cannot be compensated for orally. All oral fluids should be administered at room temperature. There is SUGGESTIVE EVIDENCE that cold fluids stimulate the gastrocolic reflex and potentiate diarrhea. Broth should not be used since it may cause hypernatremia.

Within a day or two, if the parents have administered the volumes prescribed, dehydration should no longer be a problem. Since clear fluids cannot provide adequate nutrition, it is important that the parents start feeding the infant relatively early. One of the authors has seen a number of cases of protein-calorie malnutrition in previously well-nourished middle-class infants whose parents withheld adequate nourishment because they thought that the infant could have only clear fluids until the stools became normal. In view of the fact that lactose potentiates diarrhea (4) (FIRM EVIDENCE), milk should be withheld for 4 to 5 days, but bananas, rice, biscuits, cooked potato, toast, and the like are all indicated as soon as it is clear that hydration is not compromised (usually 1 to 3 days after the diet of clear fluids is begun). The clear fluids, along with increasing amounts of solids, should be continued until the volume of stool losses decreases, as exemplified by a few bowel movements of increasing consistency. At that point, cheese that does not contain lactose (5) should be introduced into the diet, as can egg and meat, and, if all goes well, a small amount of milk. If there is no recurrence of diarrhea the volume of milk can be increased over the next few days until the regular amount is achieved. There is considerable experience (in the developing world) that indicates that breast-feeding can be resumed even within the first 24 hours of the onset of acute diarrhea as long as adequate volumes of clear fluids are also taken. For infants fed cow's milk formula in whom diarrhea recurs after milk is reinstated in the diet, 1 or 2 weeks of soybean formula may be necessary.

Opiates and opiate derivatives that slow peristalsis are not beneficial and may occasionally be harmful (6). Mixtures of kaolin and pectin are not effective and should not be used; these mixtures produce greater losses of sodium and potassium in the stools of experimental animals (FIRM EVIDENCE) (7). Attempts to colonize the intestine with lactobacilli, harmless bacteria, have no beneficial effect (FIRM EVIDENCE) (8).

CHRONIC AND RECURRENT DIARRHEA

Narrowing down

Diarrhea that persists or recurs may be classified as serious or benign. Fortunately, most children with this problem are basically healthy. The difference between the healthy ones and those with more serious causes of chronic or recurrent diarrhea lies in the observation that healthy children with "nuisance" diarrhea continue to gain weight adequately while those with more serious problems not only do not gain but may lose weight.

Serious causes of chronic diarrhea, although rare, can usually be diagnosed on the basis of the history and physical examination, with laboratory tests used to confirm the clinical impression. Such causes include cystic fibrosis, celiac disease, inflammatory bowel disease, and chronic nonspecific life-threatening diarrhea of infancy. Since many asymptomatic children are infested with parasites such as *Giardia*, it is not clear what role these organisms play in the pathogenesis of chronic or recurrent diarrhea.

Diagnosis

The healthy, growing, active infant with recurrent or chronic diarrhea generally needs no more than a careful history-taking and physical examination.

Children who do not grow adequately and who have frequent loose stools in the face of adequate caloric intake should undergo tests for cystic fibrosis, celiac disease, or other serious illnesses, as outlined in Chapter 19.

One inexpensive outpatient test that distinguishes true cow's milk protein allergy from lactose intolerance in older infants or toddlers is the following: It is known that in hard cheese all the lactose has been broken down, but it still contains cow's milk protein. If a child does not have recurrent diarrhea when given cheese but does have diarrhea when given cow's milk, it can be assumed that he or she does not have cow's milk allergy but rather cannot tolerate lactose.

In the thriving child with loose stools, laboratory tests are rarely helpful. Stool tests for ova and parasites may yield *Giardia* but should be done only if the child is not gaining weight appropriately. The selective use of laboratory tests is indicated only in cases in which positive results will have an effect on management.

Management

As mentioned earlier, in the thriving toddler or older child with a longstanding history of loose stools, pathology is rarely found or treatment required. Most parents can be reassured when they see their child's height and weight increasing in a fashion that is normal for that child in that family. Rarely are dietary manipulations necessary; if parents attempt dietary exclusions the physician should ensure that the child will continue to receive adequate nutrition. Although *Giardia* may be found in the child's stool, the recommended treatment—metronidazole, 25 mg/kg/24 hours in three doses—is oncogenic in experimental animals. Its use should therefore be limited to children with giardiasis who are not thriving. The treatment of chronic or recurrent diarrhea in nonthriving children is that of the underlying disease, for example, cystic fibrosis, celiac disease, or inflammatory bowel disease. The management of these illnesses is complicated and should be handled by consultants.

CONSTIPATION

Narrowing down

Constipation can be defined as the relatively infrequent passage of stool that is harder than normal and associated with difficulty, pain, and/or blood. Many infants and children with this problem have a family history that is positive for constipation. In fact, the concordance rate for constipation in monozygous twins is significantly greater than in dizygous twins (9). A diet inadequate in fiber may predispose the child to constipation. Medical causes of constipation in infants and children are infrequent, but they include

Hirschsprung's disease and hypothyroidism. In both, the constipation is present virtually from birth.

Acute episodes of acquired constipation may follow changes in the child's usual routine, for example, a family camping trip during which outhouses are used, or starting school, where there are strange toilet facilities. An acute episode may lead to a more chronic problem: for example, withholding of a stool because of anxiety about a strange toilet may lead to an anal fissure. Subsequent pain on defecation may result in continued withholding and chronic constipation.

Diagnosis

Laboratory tests are useful only in helping diagnose two uncommon conditions: Hirschsprung's disease (aganglionic megacolon) and hypothyroidism. In Hirschsprung's disease the constipation is virtually always present from birth; this is rarely the case in constipation from other causes. In addition, children with Hirschsprung's disease rarely have rectal bleeding or soiling. The size of the stool eventually passed is usually small; in fact, diarrhea may occur, as may malnutrition and abdominal distention. If the rectum is packed with stool, one can be reasonably certain that the child does not have Hirschsprung's disease. If there is doubt after the clinical assessment, a barium enema is indicated, which will generally show an empty segment of rectum, representing the aganglionic segment, with dilated normal ganglionic bowel above. If this disease is suspected, the child should be referred to a pediatric center for confirmation of the disease by rectal biopsy and for subsequent management.

A child with acquired hypothyroidism that causes constipation (children with congenital hypothyroidism will already have been identified in neonatal screening programs) will have growth problems, be intolerant of cold, be hypoactive, and have a slow pulse, cool skin, and other signs of hypothyroidism. The determination of serum thyroxine, thyroid stimulating hormone, and thyroid antibody levels is required to confirm the diagnosis.

Management

Constipation (as defined earlier) is rarely a problem in breast-fed, otherwise healthy, infants. Constipation usually begins once the infant starts on solid foods. In most cases, the addition of small amounts of fiber (e.g., one teaspoon of natural bran) to the infant's cereal will provide sufficient bulk. If this is not effective, another teaspoon can be added. Fruits such as prunes, either pureed or as juice, are often effective. These dietary steps can be taken when the infant is 4 to 6 months old or whenever the infant takes foods other than milk. They are also effective in older children, with increasing amounts being added on a trial-and-error basis.

For children (4 years of age and older) who balk at bran in their diet, the authors have been successful in getting many children to voluntarily increase their dietary fiber substantially with popcorn. Obviously, a proper randomized, controlled trial comparing popcorn with placebo in the treatment of childhood constipation would be difficult to conduct, but other sources of corn fiber have been studied in this way and are effective in treating what is likely a constipation-related problem (10).

If an anal fissure is seen, dietary measures may not be enough. The daily insertion of a gloved, lubricated little finger may also be required. If the infant continues to withhold stool because of pain, a topical anesthetic may be required.

Medications such as stool-softening agents (dioctyl sodium sulfosuccinate, 5 to 10 mg/kg/24 hours), senna syrup (0.5 to 3 teaspoons), mineral oil (1 to 2 ounces daily) or magnesium sulfate are rarely required and should, in uncomplicated constipation, be used only for short periods. Enemas or suppositories are indicated only in crises and should never be considered in ongoing management. Hypotonic enemas (tap water or soap) should never be used as they frequently result in water intoxication and seizures.

ACUTE ABDOMINAL PAIN

Narrowing down

Acute abdominal pain severe enough for the parents to bring the child to a physician is often caused by constipation. Abdominal cramps may be present for hours before the onset of vomiting and diarrhea in gastroenteritis. Appendicitis is a fairly common cause of acute abdominal pain, particularly in school-aged children. Acute conditions of the urinary system, such as pyelonephritis and renal colic, should also be considered, particularly if the pain is most severe in the flank and if there are other urinary symptoms. Pyelonephritis can occur at any age. Renal colic is uncommon but can be found even in preschool-aged children.

In infants, acute abdominal pain can be caused by conditions such as a strangulated inguinal hernia or intussusception. In sexually active girls, lower-quadrant pain can be the result of pelvic inflammatory disease caused by sexually transmitted organisms (see Chapter 25) or of ectopic pregnancy.

Diagnosis

Acute pain resulting from constipation can be diagnosed on the basis of a history of inadequate frequency or too-hard consistency of bowel movements, a fecal mass (usually in the left lower quadrant), and a rectal examination that demonstrates a rectum packed with feces. There will be no fever and no evidence of peritoneal irritation. The pain will be completely relieved after defecation. It may be necessary to use either a glycerin suppository or a small enema.

The child with acute appendicitis usually has nausea and/or vomiting, periumbilical pain, and usually low-grade fever. The pain soon shifts to the right lower quadrant. As peritoneal irritation increases, tenderness in the right lower quadrant becomes more severe and the child will prefer to lie perfectly still. In preschool-aged children the clinical course is often atypical and the diagnosis difficult. In general, the typical case presents few diagnostic problems. In all age groups, atypical presentations may occur, usually because the appendix in such individuals is not located in the right lower quadrant, so that the pain and tenderness may be in the hypogastrium, the flank (if retrocolic), or the pelvis. In infants, irritability and an insistence on lying supine with the hips in flexion may be the only clues to appendicitis. On occasion, an acutely inflamed appendix may irritate the adjacent colon, leading to diarrhea, or a pelvic appendix may irritate the bladder, leading to urinary urgency and frequency.

In the usual case of appendicitis, the white blood cell count is elevated to between 10,000 and 16,000 per milliliter. When acute appendicitis is suspected, urgent consultation with a surgeon skilled in dealing with children is essential, since a delay in diagnosis and treatment could lead to rupture of the appendix and serious complications.

Urinalysis and urine culture will confirm those cases in which acute abdominal pain is caused by urinary tract infection.

A kidney stone often can be suspected on clinical grounds, especially if there is a family history of stones, but urinalysis, straining of the urine for sediment, abdominal ultrasound, and an intravenous pyelogram should be considered, especially if the symptoms persist and no other cause is apparent.

Intussusception occurs most commonly between 3 months and 3 years of age and typically presents with a sudden onset of intense pain that recurs in frequent paroxysms. The child shrieks with pain, and the parents of affected children say that the cries are unlike any their children previously demonstrated. Frequently the pain is accompanied by straining. Initially the child may be quite well between paroxysms, but eventually he or she looks quite ill. At some point 60% of affected patients pass a mixture of blood and mucus, the so-called currant jelly stool. A sausage-shaped mass is palpable in the abdomen. The mass becomes more discrete during the paroxysms of pain. The rectal examination may demonstrate bloody mucus. A plain film of the abdomen or abdominal ultrasound will suggest the diagnosis. A barium enema performed by a radiologist skilled in working with children will often not only be diagnostic but, with the appropriate amount of hydrostatic pressure, be therapeutic in reducing the intussusception. If intussusception is suspected, the child should be referred to a pediatric center where skilled pediatric radiologists and surgeons are available.

Management

Acute constipation   Acute abdominal pain, severe enough to require medical attention, caused by constipation should be treated with a hypertonic phosphate enema or a glycerin suppository. The mainstay of management after the acute episode is preventive (see section on constipation above).

Acute appendicitis   The treatment for acute appendicitis is surgery.

Urinary tract infection or kidney stone   See Chapter 10.

Intussusception   A barium enema administered by a radiologist skilled in dealing with infants will actually cure the intussusception in about 75% of cases. The child should be examined by a pediatric surgeon when the diagnosis is first suspected.

BLOOD IN THE STOOLS

Narrowing down

There are two key questions that have to be asked in considering the problem of blood in the stool. The first relates to the urgency with which the diagnosis and management need to be made: How much blood has been lost? Usually parents cannot say exactly, but they will know if the blood is just a streak on the stool or if the toilet bowl or diaper is full of red blood. The second question relates to the cause of bleeding: Is defecation painful or painless? Painful defecation associated with the passage of a hard stool streaked with blood is due to constipation and either an anal fissure or hemorrhoids. Tarry, painless stools in children are due to the same causes of upper gastrointestinal bleeding as exist in adults, for example, peptic ulcer or gastroesophageal reflux leading to esophagitis. Fortunately, these conditions are uncommon. In infants, bloody stool associated with severe abdominal pain may be caused by intussusception. Bloody diarrhea, if acute, is usually due to gastroenteritis, either viral or bacterial; chronic or recurrent blood with diarrhea may be due to inflammatory bowel disease, especially if the child has recurrent abdominal pain, loses weight or appetite, becomes apathetic, and/or has recurrent fevers.

Diagnosis

If the blood in the stool is felt on the basis of the history and physical examination to be due to constipation and an anal fissure or hemorrhoids, and if the amount of blood is small and the child is thriving, no further tests need be done. If there is bloody diarrhea, and infection has been ruled out by appropriate cultures, then barium studies and referral to a pediatrician experienced in dealing with inflammatory bowel disease are indicated. Hemoglobin levels, a blood smear, and the child's iron status should be determined early on to provide baseline values, especially if the bleeding persists.

Painless bleeding of red blood, usually scanty but occasionally worrisome, indicates the need for a complete blood cell count, blood smear, iron status, and coagulation studies. At the same time, an air-barium contrast study should be done to demonstrate a colonic polyp.

Tarry stools, which represent upper gastrointestinal bleeding, indicate the need for a complete blood cell count and blood smear and urgent referral to a pediatrician experienced in handling upper gastrointestinal bleeding.

Management

The management of blood in the stools caused by constipation or infectious diarrhea is straightforward (see above sections on constipation and diarrhea). If these are ruled out, the patient should be referred to a consultant experienced in the diagnosis and management of the other much less common but potentially disastrous conditions.

FECAL SOILING (ENCOPRESIS)

Narrowing down

Fecal soiling that continues beyond the age of 4 years in children who demonstrate normal development in other spheres and in whom there are no abnormal findings on physical examination is a fairly common source of anxiety for parents. Although there are those who feel that encopresis is primarily a psychologic disorder (11), others believe it is due primarily to chronic constipation and that explanation and treatment of the constipation result in a high rate of cure, without formal psychotherapy and without evidence of symptom substitution (12).

Diagnosis

In the child whose history is suggestive of acquired megacolon (soiling, history of constipation, infrequent passage of massive stools that may clog the toilet, and otherwise normal growth and development) and in whom physical examination reveals a descending colon that is distended with feces and a dilated rectum full of feces, no laboratory tests or radiographic assessments are required.

Management

There are a number of different treatments proposed for this condition, all of which have three principles in common.

Education The child and parents must be made aware of the abnormal physiology secondary to megacolon, with resultant seepage around the constipated (retained) rectal mass. Guilt feelings should be alleviated, for both child and parents.

Evacuation Although most textbooks stress the use of enemas and suppositories in the initial phase, the authors have rarely found it necessary to recommend this form of therapy. Regular evacuation of the rectum is essential if control is to be regained, but this can be done using laxatives, usually over a 6- to 12-month period. Although mineral oil is the laxative most widely recommended, there is NO CLEAR EVIDENCE that it is more effective than the more acceptable senna laxatives such as Senekot, 1 to 3 teaspoons or tablets as necessary to result in a bowel movement in the toilet every day. The child should be encouraged (but not forced) to sit on the toilet twice each day, about 15 to 20 minutes after eating, after breakfast and after dinner, until a regular pattern develops. Some parents insist that their child sit on the toilet until he has a bowel movement, but 5 to 10 minutes is long enough; otherwise the child will view this ritual as punishment.

Follow-up The child should be examined regularly, weekly for a few weeks and then less often. The child and parent should chart the frequency of bowel movements in the toilet, as well as the frequency and amount of soiling. The dose of laxative should be adjusted accordingly. A high-fiber diet should be encouraged, especially one including sources of fiber that most children enjoy, for example, popcorn. If there are signs of improvement, the primary care physician should continue his or her management without consulting other physicians. If there is no improvement, and especially if there seems to be a large voluntary component to the soiling (e.g., it happens only when company arrives), the help of a consultant experienced in dealing with these problems should be sought.

At all times, the physician and parents should conspire to improve the child's self-esteem. Behavior modification without laxative treatment rarely works; similarly, medical management without praise for success is less likely to be effective.

REFERENCES

1. McCormick, M.C. *Epidemiology of Diarrhea in the United States.* Ross Roundtables on Critical Approaches to Common Pediatric Problems. Columbus, Oh.: Ross Laboratories, August 1982, p. 5.

2. Illingsworth, R.S. *Common Symptoms of Disease in Children*, 7th ed. Oxford: Blackwell Scientific Publications, 1982.
3. Feldman, W., Pennie, R., Ritter, H. Oral electrolyte solutions vs. unspecified clear fluids in the management of mild gastroenteritis in infants. *Am. J. Dis. Child.*, 140, 4:303, 1986(abstract).
4. Sutton, R.E., Hamilton, J.R. Tolerance of young children with severe gastroenteritis to dietary lactose: A controlled study. *Can. Med. Assoc. J.* 99:980–982, 1968.
5. De Waard, H. Lactose in yogurt (Letter). *Lancet*, 1:605, 1980.
6. Curtis, J.A., Goel, K.M. Lomotil poisoning in children. *Arch. Dis. Child.* 54:222–225, 1979.
7. McCling, M.J., Beck, R.D., Powers, P. The effect of a kaolin-pectin absorbent on stool losses of sodium, potassium and fat during a lactose-intolerance diarrhoea in rats. *J. Pediatrics* 96:769–771, 1980.
8. Pearce, J.L., Hamilton, J.R. Controlled trial of orally administered lactobacilli in acute infantile diarrhoea. *J. Pediatr.* 84:261–262, 1974.
9. Bakwin, H., Davidson, M. Constipation in twins. *Am. J. Dis. Child.* 121:179–181, 1971.
10. Feldman, W., McGrath, P., Hodgson, C., Ritter, H., Shipman, R.T. The use of dietary fibre in the management of simple childhood idiopathic recurrent abdominal pain: Results in a prospective double blind randomized controlled trial. *Am. J. Dis. Child.* 139:1216–1218, 1985.
11. Behrman, R.E., Vaughan, V.C. III, eds. Nelson, Textbook of Pediatrics. Philadelphia: W.B. Saunders, 1983, p. 74.
12. Levine, M.P., Mazonson, P., Bakow, H. Behavioural symptom substitution in children cured of encopresis. *Am. J. Dis. Child.* 134:663–667, 1980.

6

SKIN PROBLEMS

Skin problems are extremely common in children, from birth throughout childhood. Almost every child will be afflicted with some type of dermatitis during his or her first 5 years of life.

This chapter is organized somewhat differently from the others in that it is divided into three sections, by age group: birth to 1 year, 1 to 5 years, and 5 to 18 years. These represent three phases of childhood in which there are different common skin conditions. Infants often have skin conditions related to contact with diaper or clothing. Preschool-aged children suffer different skin conditions than do school-aged children. To assist the clinician in narrowing down the causes of skin lesions, the skin conditions have been divided into two categories; those that are and those that are not accompanied by systemic illness. The thorough physician will assess first the general condition of the child, second, the distribution of the rash, and, finally, the characteristics of the rash.

Tables 6-1 through 6-5 are designed to assist in determining the most likely causes of rashes in children. Reference to a detailed pediatric or dermatology textbook will be necessary for the less common conditions.

BIRTH TO 1 YEAR

Prevalence

Staphylococcal scalded skin syndrome is, fortunately, very rare in newborns; it occurs no more than once in several thousand births. Toxic erythema of the newborn is seen in approximately 50% of all newborns, usually on the second or third day of life. Livedo neonatorum is seen in virtually every newborn if the skin becomes cool. Milia occur in 10 to 20% of newborn babies and increase in intensity up to 6 weeks and then fade by 3 months. Hemangiomas are seen in approximately 10% of infants in the first 4 to 6 weeks of life.

Table 6-1. Skin diseases with systemic effects in infants from birth to 1 year

Whole-body distribution			Focal distribution	
Erythematous macules	Bullae	Congenital abnormalities	Papules	Macules
Staphylococcal scalded skin syndrome* Toxic erythema of the newborn*	Pemphigus neonatorum	Pigmentary diseases Glycogen and lipid storage diseases Neurofibromatosis Ichthyosis	Sclerema neonatorum	Impetigo neonatorum

*Condition described in the text.

Narrowing down and diagnosis: Conditions with systemic effects

Scalded skin syndrome Although rare, scalded skin syndrome is mentioned here because it rapidly becomes life-threatening if not detected early. Scalded skin syndrome is caused by a staphylococcal systemic infection and is characterized by a high fever (39°C) accompanied by widespread erythema and bullae. A positive Nikolsky's sign (the separation of epidermis in response to gentle stroking) is diagnostic.

Narrowing down: Conditions without systemic effects

Toxic erythema of the newborn Toxic erythema of the newborn usually appears in an asymptomatic, vigorous, and hungry infant on the second or third day of life. Most of the lesions are urticarial and erythematous, some are papular; they appear anywhere on the body. The lesions become confluent and usually disappear spontaneously within 4 to 5 days. The main task of the physician is to reassure the parents that the condition is completely benign and will disappear spontaneously.

Table 6-2. Skin diseases without systemic effects in infants from birth to 1 year

Whole-body distribution	Focal distribution
Toxic erythema of the newborn* Livedo neonatorum* Carotenemia	Milia* Hemangiomas* Herpes simplex*

*Condition described in the text.

Livedo neonatorum In livedo neonatorum, the skin becomes mottled with a bluish discoloration anywhere on the body, usually when the child is cool. The cause is not well understood but is probably secondary to instability of the sympathetic nervous system, which controls blood circulation to the skin. Children who are more prone to mottling may experience episodes even when the skin is warm, up to the age of 1 year, at which time the problem disappears. Reassuring the parents that the condition is benign is important.

Milia Milia appear at birth as tiny white papules, usually on the face, and increase in number and intensity up to about 6 weeks of age. They usually completely disappear within 3 months. Their appearance on the infant's face often distresses the parents. Reassuring the parents that these lesions will completely disappear is the physician's role. There is NO CLEAR EVIDENCE that any therapy is effective.

Hemangiomas Hemangiomas evident at birth can be strawberry hemangiomata, which tend to be erythematous and raised above the skin surface, or benign hemangiomas, which tend to become confluent with the skin and are essentially a purplish discoloration. Both types of hemangiomas may increase in size in the first 6 months of life but usually fade by age 5. Treatment of hemangiomata is required only if the lesion compresses a vital structure, such as the eye, in which case referral to a specialist is required. Otherwise, patience on the part of parents and the physician is all that is necessary.

1 TO 5 YEARS

Prevalence

The increasing numbers of children attending day-care centers has resulted in a rising incidence of infectious diseases in the 1- to 5-year-old age group. Urticaria is a relatively infrequent problem in this age group but varies with diet, climate, and the sensitivity of the population. Insect bites are common in infants, with the incidence varying according to climate, time of year, and humidity; socioeconomic conditions also influence the incidence and type of insect bites. Systemic reactions to insect bites, usually of bees, occur in 0.4% of the population. The incidence of scabies increases if hygiene and living conditions are poor. Warts or verrucae vulgaris may be seen in up to 20% of children.

Contact dermatitis occurs in virtually all infants, especially those under 2 who wear diapers. Eczema occurs in approximately 10% of children under age 5. Significant seborrheic dermatitis is seen in 10 to 20% of babies, most commonly in the first 18 months of life. With the current immunization programs, infectious diseases such as rubella and rubeola have become uncom-

Table 6-3. Skin diseases without systemic effects in children 1 to 5 years old

Whole-body distribution		Focal distribution		
Papular	Macular	Papular	Maculopapular	Other

Herpes simplex*	Urticaria*
	Erythema
	  infectiosum
		Bites*
		Scabies*
		Verrucae
		  vulgaris*
		Juvenile warts*
		Molluscum
		  contagiosum*
		Pityriasis
		  rubra pilaris
		Juvenile
		  melanoma
			Contact
			  dermatitis*
			Eczema*
			Seborrhea*
			Folliculitis
				Bruising
				Cat scratch
				  fever
				Tenia
				  infections
				Vitiligo

*Condition described in the text.

mon. Approximately 10 to 20% of infants under 2 years of age suffer from roseola infantum, while varicella is the most common infectious skin disease in the 4- to 8-year age group, affecting up to 90%. Impetigo and herpes simplex are common, but their frequency varies according to hygiene and the degree of exposure to others who are infected.

Narrowing down: Conditions without systemic effects

Urticaria   Urticarial lesions are usually generalized; they occur anywhere on the body, and come and go within minutes to hours. The lesions are usually raised and warm, and may be light red or have erythema around an area of central pallor. Urticaria may be caused by a wide range of foods. In fewer than half of all cases is a specific cause found; the foods most commonly incriminated are strawberries, raspberries, and nuts. Products containing food coloring have also been implicated. In most cases urticaria resolves spontaneously.

Insect bites   Parents should take precautions to prevent their children from bites by flying insects during the summer, especially in more tropical climates where reactions to bites may be more severe than in northern areas. There is a less-than-1% risk of anaphylactic reactions to the bites of bees and other stinging insects. Insect bites are always discrete, generally multiple, and lesions are usually papillary. The stinger or point of entry of the sting may be visible at the center of the lesion. Bee stings may produce allergic anaphylaxis in addition to severe local reactions, such as a large wheal and flare. Anaphylaxis may result in upper and lower airway obstruction and symptoms of peripheral vascular collapse.

Scabies   In children who do not practice good hygiene, scabies is relatively common. Lesions are often seen between the fingers or on the arms, but the lesions may occur on the legs or anywhere on the body. The lesions are extremely pruritic. The erythematous tracks of the tiny mites can be seen on careful assessment using magnification.

Verrucae vulgaris (warts)   Verucae vulgaris are more common in older children but may occur in any age group. Warts are characterized by a circumscribed raised papilla, usually with a rough cauliflowerlike surface that is often cracked. Removal of the surface will reveal the characteristic blackened blood vessels that enter the root of the lesion. Verrucae vulgaris usually spontaneously remit even if they have persisted for many years. The virus that causes these lesions is moderately infectious.

Juvenile warts   Juvenile warts are usually seen in clusters of six to eight, are slightly raised macular lesions without discoloration, and are confluent with the skin. They often occur on the skin of face, arms, or back.

Molloscum contagiosum   Molluscum contagiosum is characterized by small (1 to 5 millimeters) papular lesions with a punctate central area. The lesions are caused by a virus and treatment consists of benign neglect, since they are often self-limited and resolve in 6 months to 1 year.

Contact dermatitis   Diaper-wearing infants are prone to diaper dermatitis. Many theories have been put forward as to why the lesions are so common. It is believed that bacterial breakdown of the urea in urine takes place inside the warm diaper, producing ammonia that irritates the skin in an environment that also promotes the growth of *Candida albicans*. The skin-folds of the gluteal region provide other dark, warm areas for monilial growth. *Candida* infection, often originating from the stool, leads to skin breakdown and erythematous, "punched out" ulcers. Monilial superinfection is associated with redness in the skin-folds and small satellite lesions. In simple contact diaper dermatitis, the skin-folds are protected and are not involved in the dermatitis.

Eczema (atopic dermatitis)   Eczematous lesions are common in infants and children. Characteristically, lesions occur in the antecubital and popliteal fossae, and around the ears and face. However, lesions may occur at any site on the body. Eczema is characterized by erythematous lesions that often ooze serosanguinous exudates that cause considerable scaling. Lesions usually begin as erythematous patches and evolve into very pruritic lesions.

Seborrhea   The scale of seborrheic dermatitis is often seen on the eyelids or the forehead of infants. There may be a build-up of scale in the scalp causing ugly, large, yellowish patches. The hallmark of seborrhea is the dry, scaly, erythematous, papular nonpruritic lesion. Seborrhea may involve the face, the neck, the skin behind the ears, the axillae, and, quite often, the diaper area. On the extremities the lesions may resemble those of eczema but they are not pruritic.

Bruising Bruising in a child between the ages of 1 and 5 years suggests two significant problems that necessitate careful investigation. It is common for active children, aged 1 to 5, to have multiple bruises on the legs because of frequent falls, but bruising in any other area should be viewed as particularly suggestive of child abuse (see Table 14-5). The history will not always be helpful in sorting out the cause of bruising if child abuse is the problem. The second major cause of bruising is coagulation problems such as idiopathic thrombocytopenic purpura. Leukemia may be present if there is a tendency to bruise. Bruises mainly below the waist suggest Schönlein-Henoch purpura, especially if there is joint and/or abdominal pain. An unusual amount or location of bruising suggests a serious coagulation problem or abuse, and should prompt an urgent consultation to the appropriate individual or child abuse assessment team.

Narrowing down: Conditions with systemic effects

Rubella Most children have now been immunized against rubella by age 15 months (see Table 14-2). The rubelliform rash is an extensive, fine, papular rash that blanches on compression and is most concentrated in the truncal region, with lesser extension to the arms and face. Usually the child develops coryza for 2 or 3 days accompanied by a low-grade fever. Usually, the postauricular or suboccipital lymph nodes are enlarged and painful. The rash may appear spontaneously, with no systemic effects, and pass within 3 or 4 days. The illness is often so mild that it is not brought to the attention of a

Table 6-4. Skin diseases with systemic effects in children 1 to 5 years old

Whole-body distribution			Focal distribution	
Papular	Macular	Other	Papular	Macular
Rubella*	Scarlatinal	Stevens-	Erythema	Impetigo*
Rubeola*	rash	Johnson	nodosum	Herpes
Roseola	Atopic	syndrome		simplex*
infantum*	erythroderma	Schönlein-		Erysipelas
Varicella*	Pityriasis	Henoch		Erythema
Viral exanthema	rosea	purpura*		multiforme

*Condition described in the text.

physician. There is no treatment, but extreme caution about rubella exposure to pregnant women, especially those in the first trimester, must be exercised. Rubella during the first weeks of pregnancy leads to a 50% rate of congenital rubella syndrome in the newborn (see Chapter 14).

Rubeola After two decades of extensive immunization programs, which in many jurisdictions are now required by law for children before they enter school, rubeola has become a relatively rare disease. It is usually accompanied by severe systemic symptoms, characterized by a 3- to 4- day prodromal phase of high fever, coryza, conjunctivitis, and pharyngitis. Accompanying the high fever during the first 2 to 3 days of the rash are photophobias and Koplik's spots. The erythematous macular rash is very dense over the face and truncal areas but usually less so over the extremities. Twenty percent of afflicted children develop pneumonitis or otitis media. There is no effective therapeutic intervention available other than symptomatic treatment. Because of the past use of killed-measles vaccine, atypical rubeola may occur but it is rare.

Roseola infantum Roseola infantum starts with a high temperature of between 39 and 41°C, lasting approximately 48 hours. When the temperature drops to normal, an extensive papular rash appears. Roseola infantum presents a diagnostic dilemma during the febrile phase when no rash is present, since on physical examination there are no findings to explain the fever. The physician may be tempted to prescribe an antibiotic. When the temperature drops within 24 hours and a rash appears, then the dilemma arises of whether to attribute the rash to antibiotic allergies. Children in the 12-month to 3-year-old age group who have high fever and no focal physical findings are probably best managed by re-examination every 12 to 24 hours (see Chapter 1).

Varicella With more children exposed to other children at a younger age in day-care centers, the highest incidence of varicella has begun to shift to the preschool-aged group. Varicella is characterized mainly by a truncal rash of macules, papules, vesicles, and crusts. The accompanying systemic illness is usually mild, except in infants and adults. The prodrome is a low-grade fever (38 to 39°C) for 24 to 48 hours preceding the appearance of the rash. Occasionally vesicles in the mouth coexist with or antedate the skin lesions. The incubation period is usually 14 to 18 days from exposure to the onset of the rash. Many parents apply calamine lotion to the lesions in an attempt to reduce the pruritis. Parents should be advised against using calamine lotion because the talc in the lotion may rarely produce talc granuloma, resulting in permanent scars. Application of cold cloths for topical pruritis is usually effective, and may be assisted by the administration of antihistamines such is diphenhydramine, 5 mg/kg/24 hours in three doses.

Impetigo Impetigo is a common skin infection usually caused by Group A beta-hemolytic streptococci. Systemic penicillin combined with topical treatment by frequently washing the crusting lesions, is appropriate. The condition is characterized by a mucopurulent exudate that forms and rapidly spreads over the face or other areas of the body. Impetigo is readily transmitted between individuals; the steps to control its spread include washing the hands and boiling hand-towels, facecloths, and other contaminated or potentially contaminated materials.

Herpes simplex Herpes simplex lesions are less common than impetigo in this age group but must be differentiated from the early stages of impetigo. The lesions begin with a characteristic maculopapular cluster of lesions that blister and may become confluent in ulcers. The lesions appear anywhere on the skin surface. No satisfactory therapy exists. The lesions heal within 10 to 14 days after the first appearance of macules.

5 TO 18 YEARS

Narrowing down

Tables 6-5 and 6-6 outline the common skin problems, both without and with systemic effects, in children aged 5 to 18. See the previous section for descriptions of the skin conditions; those that occur in children aged 1 to 5 continue to show up in the 5- to 18-year age group. See Chapter 25 for information about acne vulgaris.

Table 6-5. Skin diseases without systemic effects in children 5 to 18 years old

Whole-body distribution		Focal distribution		
Papular	Macular	Papular	Macular	Other
Herpes simplex*	Urticaria*	Bites*	Contact	Bruising
	Pityriasis	Scabies*	dermatitis*	Tinea
	rosea	Acne vulgaris*	Seborrheic	Vitiligo
		Verruca	dermatitis*	Alopecia
		vulgaris*	Psoriasis	
		Molluscum	Folliculitis	
		contagiosum*		
		Acne rosacea		
		Furunculosis		
		Pityriasis		
		rubra pilaris		

*Condition described in the text.

Table 6-6. Skin diseases with systemic effects in children 5 to 18 years old

Whole-body distribution			Focal distribution	
Papular	Macular	Other	Papular	Macular
Rubella*	Scarlatinal	Stevens-	Erythema	Erysipelas
Rubeola*	rash	Johnson	nodosum	Erythema
Varicella*	Atopic	syndrome		Impetigo*
Viral exanthema	erythroderma	Schönlein-		
		Henoch		
		purpura		

*Condition described in the text.

MANAGEMENT OF SKIN PROBLEMS FOR WHICH EFFECTIVE TREATMENT EXISTS

Staphylococcal scalded skin syndrome   Scalded skin syndrome should be treated in the hospital. Intravenous antistaphylococcal antibiotics, such as cloxacillin, 100 mg/kg/24 hours in divided doses, are associated with excellent results. If the infant is drinking well and is not in a toxic condition, a trial of oral cloxacillin in the same dose can be attempted first. Because of the life-threatening nature of this illness, if there is no significant improvement in 24 to 48 hours, consultation with a specialist is recommended.

Urticaria   A food diary should be kept in an attempt to determine the causative agent of urticaria. Obviously, if specific foods are consistently associated with symptoms, they should be avoided. For relief of the itch, diphenhydramine, 5 mg/kg/24 hours in three doses, or hydroxyzine, 2 mg/kg/24 hours in three doses, may be administered. If this does not suffice and the itch is very uncomfortable, epinephrine, 0.2 to 0.3 milliliters subcutaneously will generally provide rapid relief.

Severe reactions to insect bites   In an anaphylactic reaction to a bee sting, the administration of epinephrine 1:1,000, 0.2–0.3 milliliters subcutaneously, may be life-saving. If peripheral vascular collapse occurs, blood volume expanders may also be necessary. Intravenous diphenhydramine (25 to 50 milligrams) may also be used, but there is NO CLEAR EVIDENCE that it is effective. Kits containing a syringe with epinephrine and an antihistamine tablet should be available to parents of children who have had a severe local or systemic reaction. These children should wear a Medic-Alert bracelet. There is FIRM EVIDENCE that children who have airway or blood pressure problems after insect bites and a positive skin test should have specific immunotherapy (1). Immunotherapy is not mandatory if the lesions are only cutaneous.

Scabies   The drug of choice for scabies is 1% gamma benzene hexachloride, even though it is neurotoxic when ingested (2). Infants under 1 year of age may experience neurotoxicity with the usual duration of application of the cream or lotion (8 to 12 hours over the whole body, from the neck down). A shorter application, 6 hours, is recommended for them. There is NO CLEAR EVIDENCE that traditional treatments, such as crotamiton cream or 6% sulfur, are less toxic or more effective for infants less than 6 months old (3).

Warts   Since most warts disappear on their own with time, they can usually be ignored. If they are very unsightly, salicylic acid (10 to 17%) in collodion may be applied daily. Plantar warts can be treated with 40% salicylic acid plasters, but they will usually recur until they resolve spontaneously. They should be treated only if there is pain on walking. Liquid nitrogen or salicylic acid should be used with extreme caution on the face: a wart will eventually disappear without any treatment but a scar from treatment will not. A consultation with a dermatologist is suggested if a child has unsightly facial warts.

Molluscum contagiosum   Since the lesions of molluscum contagiosum are usually self-limited, the only indications for treatment are the spread of lesions from one site to another or the possibility of the spread of the disease to other children, for instance, in a day-care center. The lesions will disappear if the central core is removed using a needle (4).

Contact dermatitis   If a skin rash is clearly related to wearing a watch band, new shoes, or other obvious irritant, then removal of the specific irritant will result in a cure. For diaper dermatitis, diapers should be changed frequently and the diaper area exposed to air. The area should be cleaned with warm water but without soap. If a monilial infection appears to be superimposed on the diaper dermatitis, application of Mycostatin cream, or, if severe, a combination of Mycostatin and 1% hydrocortisone cream, should result in marked improvement. For resistant monilial diaper dermatitis, oral Mycostatin has been recommended, but there is NO CLEAR EVIDENCE that it is superior to topical therapy (5). After the diaper dermatitis clears, occlusive elastic-legged pants should not be worn. Application of zinc oxide paste (1%) or corn starch may prevent recurrence.

Eczema (atopic dermatitis)   The role of diet is controversial in eczema, but there is NO CLEAR EVIDENCE that specific diets are beneficial. If parents observe a flare-up after the child eats specific foods, they should withhold these foods for several weeks; if there is improvement in the eczema, the foods should be reintroduced. If the skin condition then worsens, the food should be avoided for months, unless it is nutritionally essential. Before milk is removed from the diet, several trials of its removal should made because soybean substitutes are expensive.

Since perspiration irritates eczema, excessively warm and humid environments should be avoided and the child should not be overdressed. Wool clothing aggravates the condition in many children. Irritating soaps should be avoided; warm water baths may be adequate for hygiene.

Local topical therapy, such as 0.5 to 1.0% hydrocortisone cream, is the most important component of treatment. If the itch is severe, diphenhydramine, 5 mg/kg/24 hours, or hydroxyzine, 2 mg/kg/24 hours, can be prescribed.

Seborrhea The scaly scalp lesions of seborrhea may be softened and loosened with bland oil. There is NO CLEAR EVIDENCE that expensive perfumed baby oils are more effective than inexpensive vegetable oils. The softened scales can then be washed off using a bland soap. Inflamed skin lesions respond well to topical steroid therapy. Children with seborrhea often continue to have problems as adults. As they get older, commercially available antidandruff shampoos often control the scalp lesions.

REFERENCES

1. Hunt, K.J., Valentine, M.D., Sobotka, A.K., Benton, A.W., Amodia, F.J., Lichtenstein, C.M. A controlled trial of immunotherapy in insect hypersensitivity. *N. Engl. J. Med.* 299:157–161. 1978.
2. Schater, B. Treatment of scabies and pediculosis with lindane preparations. *J. Am. Acad. Dermatol.* 5:517–527, 1981.
3. Rasmussen, J.E. The problem of lindane. *J. Am. Acad. Dermatol.* 5:507–516. 1981.
4. Tunnessen, W.W., Cutaneous infections. *Pediatr. Clin. North Am.* 30:515–532. 1983.
5. Munz, D., Powell, K., Dal, C. Treatment of candidal diaper dermatitis–A double blind placebo controlled comparison of nystatin with topical plus oral nystatin. *J. Pediatr.* 101:1022–1025, 1982.

7

LOWER RESPIRATORY PROBLEMS

Lower respiratory problems (arbitrarily defined as those due to pathology in the respiratory system from the epiglottis to the alveoli) may have symptoms and signs that vary from mild to severe and last from hours to months. The major manifestations include cough, noisy breathing, and tachypnea. The relative prominence of these signs and symptoms is related to age, site of pathology, etiologic agent(s), and severity of the process.

PREVALENCE

The common causes of lower respiratory problems in children are infectious agents and asthma. Cystic fibrosis and aspiration of foreign bodies are much less common. The prevalences of the major infections (1) are, for all children, 134 in 1,000; for, infants less than 1 year old, 240 in 1,000; and for adolescents, 34 in 1,000. Most of these infections are manifested clinically as croup, bronchiolitis, and pneumonia; the younger the child is, the more likely the illness is due to a virus, especially in winter.

The prevalence of asthma in children aged 6 to 16 is 46 in 1,000 (2). Thus, if one adds the prevalence of the infectious causes of lower respiratory problems (134 in 1,000) to those of asthma (46 in 1,000) and some of the severe chronic chest conditions, at least 18% of children will at some point have an illness with the signs and symptoms of lower respiratory tract disease. The average annual number of admissions for each diagnosis in one children's hospital is shown in Table 7-1. Some children, for example, those with asthma or cystic fibrosis, are often admitted more than once each year.

This chapter deals with those lower respiratory problems that are highly prevalent (infections, asthma). In addition, some of the problems that are less prevalent (epiglottitis, foreign body aspiration) are discussed because a high awareness of such problems on the part of the family physician may save a child's life.

Table 7-1. Annual number of hospitalizations* for lower respiratory conditions

Rank order	Diagnosis	Annual number admissions
1	Asthma	658
2	Bronchiolitis	221
3	Pneumonia	217
4	Croup	189
5	Pertussis	60
6	Cystic fibrosis	36
7	Epiglottitis	17
8	Foreign body aspiration	1 every 2 years

*Mean annual admission rate at the Children's Hospital of Eastern Ontario, 1979–1983.

NARROWING DOWN

The key features necessary to help narrow down the causes of cough, noisy breathing, and tachypnea are shown in Table 7-2.

Cough as the predominant feature

A cough with serous rhinitis and no evidence of distress that lasts a week or so is usually due to a viral upper respiratory infection; it is dealt with in Chapter 2. A paraxysmal cough, possibly associated with vomiting and/or a whoop that lasts weeks to months is most often due to pertussis or a pertussislike syndrome. When it occurs for the first time, a cough in infancy that is associated with wheezing, tachypnea, and in-drawing of breath is usually bronchiolitis due mainly to respiratory syncytial virus. Recurrent episodes of this nature in otherwise healthy infants and children are usually due to asthma. A chronic or recurrent cough without wheezing in healthy children whose height and weight are progressing according to familial patterns, and which is exacerbated by exercise or cold air, is usually due to a mild variant of asthma. A chronic or recurrent cough in a child with poor growth and repeated episodes of pneumonia may be due to cystic fibrosis, immune deficiency problems, or other rare entities, such as alpha-one antitrypsin deficiency. If the pneumonia occurs consistently in the same area of the lung, foreign body aspiration or a congenital anomaly such as lobar sequestration must be considered.

A croupy cough, that is, a barking cough that sounds somewhat like the cry of a seal, is usually due to laryngotracheobronchitis, most often caused by parainfluenza virus. In healthy children, a daytime cough, that is, a cough that disappears during sleep, is usually a "habit cough," a form of tic, analogous to eye-blinking.

Table 7-2. Symptoms and signs of lower respiratory problems

Possible cause	Key features
Pertussis	Paroxymal cough with or without whoop, vomiting at end of cough; appears well between coughing spasms; worsens at night
Bronchiolitis	Respiratory distress; tachypnea; high-pitched rhonchi, mainly expiratory; occurs mainly in infants
Asthma	Improves with bronchodilator; key features same as those for bronchiolitis, but they recur
Foreign body aspiration	Acute onset; history of sudden cough and choking; hyperresonance and decreased air entry on affected side
Cystic fibrosis	Failure-to-thrive; family history; recurrent pneumonia; chronic cough; diarrhea
Croup	More in the first few years; continues to drink well; barking cough; may be in respiratory distress
Epiglottitis	Barking cough; respiratory distress; refuses to drink or swallow; patients usually older than those with croup
"Habit" cough	Thrives; cough disappears with sleep
Pneumonia	In infants, as in bronchiolitis; signs may be more localized; high fever and white blood cell count in older children suggest pneumococci

Noisy breathing as the predominant feature

Inspiratory stridor is usually due to laryngotracheobronchitis, epiglottitis, or a foreign body in the trachea or bronchus. In infants (first episode), expiratory wheezing is most often due to bronchiolitis and, in infants and older children, when recurrent, to asthma. The presence of a foreign body in a bronchus is a rare but life-threatening condition. Inspiratory stridor with croupy cough in an infant who continues to drink well is most likely caused by viral "croup." The same findings in an infant or older child who drools, refuses to drink, and looks to be in a toxic condition may well be due to epiglottitis, an infection caused by *Haemophilus influenzae* type b. An acute episode of inspiratory stridor, cough, dyspnea, cyanosis, and choking may be caused by a foreign body in the trachea.

Wheezing that is due to viral bronchiolitis occurs mainly in infants; it peaks at the age of 6 months and occurs mainly in the winter. There may be other family members who demonstrate evidence of viral respiratory infections. If bronchiolar obstruction is mild, the child may manifest only a cough, wheezing, and slight tachypnea. If the obstruction is severe, signs of respiratory distress, such as flaring of the alae nasi, suprasternal, intercostal, and substernal retractions, and cyanosis, as well as tachycardia and tachypnea, may be observed. The degree of fever is variable; temperatures as high as 39.5°C do not necessarily imply a bacterial etiology.

Recurrent episodes of wheezing may be triggered by viral infections, exercise, cold air, or inhaled allergens. It is common (and wrong) for children with such episodes to be given multiple courses of antibiotics. Most have lower airways hyperreactivity (asthma) to one or more of the above-mentioned stimuli, and they generally respond well to appropriate bronchodilator therapy.

Tachypnea as the predominant feature

Tachypnea may be due to a viral or bacterial infection of the airways, hyperreactivity of the lower airways, or foreign body aspiration. Other causes include metabolic acidemia, such as may occur in gastroenteritis, diabetic ketoacidosis, or salicylate poisoning. Congestive heart failure is, fortunately, an uncommon cause of tachypnea in children.

Tachypnea without wheezing is usually the result of viral or bacterial pneumonia, but wheezing may be present in both of these conditions. Infants and children with bacterial pneumonia may often look toxic more than the degree of respiratory distress would suggest. They usually have fever and cough, and the physical examination suggests local or patchy areas of lung involvement. Children with unexplained fever and tachypnea should undergo chest radiography because at times the auscultation and percussion findings may be negligible.

A history of diarrhea and vomiting, or polyuria, polydipsia, and weight loss, will usually suggest the metabolic causes of tachypnea. Heart failure as a cause of rapid respirations is usual associated with a history of growth problems, cyanosis, heart murmurs, or other stigmata of congenital or acquired heart disease. Fortunately, rheumatic fever is now rare in the developed world, and carditis as the sole major manifestation of rheumatic fever is uncommon.

DIAGNOSIS

Pertussis

The clinical history, along with listening to the paroxysmal cough and observing the child during and between coughing spells, is usually sufficient to diagnose pertussis. Suction of the nasopharynx for culture of the organism is usually not necessary. Other laboratory tests such as a complete blood cell count and chest radiography are usually not indicated. If there is tachypnea between paroxysms, a chest film should be made, since uncomplicated pertussis does not lead to tachypnea.

The pertussislike syndrome is probably a misnomer. Although adenovirus is occasionally isolated, its role in the pathogenesis of the disease is unclear. There is significant variability in the ability of microbiology laboratories to identify *Bordetella pertussis*. The diagnosis of "pertussislike syndrome" is made more often in communities where the laboratory is rarely successful in culturing *B. pertussis*, probably for technical reasons.

Asthma

Children who are growing well but who have recurrent, reversible lower airways disease have asthma. This condition can almost always be diagnosed without recourse to blood, radiographic, allergy, or pulmonary function tests. In older children in whom the results of the clinical examination are equivocal or whose response to management is unsatisfactory, chest films and pulmonary function measurements before and after bronchodilator therapy are helpful. Exercise provocation showing reduced forced expiratory volume that is reversed by inhaled bronchodilator is also helpful on occasion.

Serious chronic lower respiratory tract disease

Children with cystic fibrosis or other uncommon but serious chronic respiratory diseases generally are less active and demonstrate poor growth, persistent tachypnea and labored breathing, radiographic abnormalities, and possibly clubbing of the fingers or toes and cyanosis. These children should be referred to a pediatric specialist for full assessment.

Croup

The infant or young child who has the clinical manifestations of croup, is in no or moderate distress, and is drinking well does not need to undergo soft-tissue radiography of the neck to rule out the more serious, life-threatening epiglottitis. In fact, whether in the hospital or not, there are few laboratory tests required to diagnose or manage croup. Arterial blood gas tests should be performed if the child with croup is in severe distress.

Epiglottitis

It is not the degree of respiratory distress that is the early clue to the diagnosis of epiglottitis but rather drooling or inability to swallow. Children with this condition need expert pediatric intensive care urgently. Diagnostic tests such as lateral radiographs of the neck to demonstrate the swollen epiglottis should not be performed if they will delay such care. Blood cultures and a complete blood cell count as well as blood gas determinations should not be done if these tests will delay appropriate intervention by specialists. Such tests may be useful once therapy is begun.

Pneumonia

Infants with pneumonia may resemble those with bronchiolitis. If there is cough, tachypnea, fever, toxicity, and localized chest auscultatory findings, pneumonia is likely but should be confirmed with a chest radiograph. Occasionally, specific radiographic signs suggest etiologic agents, for example, staphylococcal pneumonia, that require treatment with specific antibiotics. Staphylococcal pneumonia is usually unilateral and most often is associated with pleural effusion or empyema. Pneumatoceles, that is, air-fluid levels within the consolidation are common. *Chlamydia trachomatis* may cause pneumonia, particularly in infants of about 6 weeks of age; the pneumonia is characterized by tachypnea, cough, and diffuse rales. Fever or systemic signs are often absent. The chest radiograph shows diffuse interstitial and patchy alveolar infiltrates.

In older children in whom pneumonia is suspected, chest radiographs may also suggest the etiology. Lobar consolidation becomes more prevalent in pneumococcal pneumonia as children get older. Diffuse infiltrates, particularly in the perihilar regions, suggest a viral cause. Mycoplasmal pneumonia peaks in children aged 10 to 15 years, has no specific clinical or radiographic characteristics, and requires a cold agglutinin titer of 1:64 or greater for the diagnosis.

MANAGEMENT

Specific treatments are shown in Table 7-3.

Pertussis

There is no specific treatment for pertussis. Antitussives and decongestants have not been shown to be effective (3). Antibiotics do not affect the clinical course (FIRM EVIDENCE) (3), but erythromycin given orally in a dose of 40 mg/kg/day for 5 to 7 days helps eradicate the organism and thereby shortens the period of infectivity (FIRM EVIDENCE) (4). Pertussis immune globulin does not alter the course of disease (FIRM EVIDENCE) (5). Uncontrolled studies suggest that prophylactic antibiotics may prevent pertussis in exposed siblings (SUGGESTIVE EVIDENCE) (6).

Infants aged 6 months or younger may have severe manifestations of the disease such as vomiting with dehydration and malnutrition, apnea, or cyanosis; death from pertussis, although rare, is most likely to occur in this age group (FIRM EVIDENCE) (7). Thus, most infants should be hospitalized for several days of observation, with particular attention paid to nutrition and the frequency and severity of paroxysms, as well as the ability of the infant to continue to breathe spontaneously afterward. If the condition is not severe,

Table 7-3. Management of lower respiratory problems

Cause	Management
Pertussis	Under 6 months, admit for 2–3 days' observation; feed frequently, monitor weight; give erythromycin to prevent spread
Bronchiolitis	Mild cases managed at home; if tachypnea, admit; oxygen therapy, watch nutrition and hydration
Asthma	If infrequent oral and/or inhaled bronchodilator at premonitory signs; otherwise, daily prophylaxis
Foreign body aspiration	Chest film; bronchoscopic removal
Cystic fibrosis	Sweat test; ongoing management should be handled by a cystic fibrosis clinic
Croup	Humidity if no respiratory distress; otherwise, admit and give oxygen therapy
Epiglottitis	Admit; immediate nasotracheal intubation; intravenous ampicillin and chloramphenicol
"Habit" cough	If stress on child not inordinate, reassure child and parents; encourage parents to ignore cough
Pneumonia	Radiograph very helpful; if clinical and radiographic findings suggest bacterial origin, give antibiotic; if respiratory distress, admit and give oxygen therapy

the parents are competent, and the family lives near a hospital equipped for pediatric intensive care, the infant can be discharged.

If the care of the infant or older child is to be managed at home, the parents should be instructed to feed the patient in small, frequent feedings to compensate for the fluid and nutritional losses associated with frequent emesis. In addition, they should be instructed to call the physician if they tire from lack of a sleep; brief hospitalization of the patient may be necessary for the parents' physical and mental health.

Bronchiolitis

Infants with signs of moderate to severe respiratory distress due to bronchiolitis should be hospitalized and given oxygen sufficient to keep arterial PO_2 between 80 and 100 mm Hg. If the infant is not able to feed properly, intravenous fluids are required. Salbutamol inhalant has been used, but no properly executed randomized controlled trial with sufficient sample size has been conducted (8). Steroids have been shown to be ineffective (FIRM EVIDENCE) (9). Antitussives and antihistamines are contraindicated because they may depress respiration and dry mucus. If signs of respiratory distress do not abate and the PO_2 does not improve with oxygen therapy, the infant should be transferred to a pediatric intensive care unit.

The care of infants with only slight tachypnea but no retractions or flaring of the alae nasi, who continue to smile and to feed well, can be managed at home. There should be daily telephone contact between physician and parents, and the parents should be instructed to call if symptoms worsen. No medications are indicated and there is NO CLEAR EVIDENCE that the use of a humidifier is helpful.

Asthma

Children in whom asthma attacks occur once every 2 months or more often should be given chronic maintenance therapy. Theophylline, 20 mg/kg/day, can be safely administered to most children (SUGGESTIVE EVIDENCE) (10). To increase compliance, the slow-release granules need be given only twice a day in children who cannot swallow slow-release tablets or capsules. In children whose attacks are less frequent, theophylline in the same dosage can be given at the first sign that an attack is imminent: running nose, cough, irritability. There is almost always a 24-hour period of premonitory signs that will signal the need for early therapy to prevent wheezing. In children whose only manifestation of asthma is a chronic or recurrent cough, and if the cough is troublesome, maintenance therapy at the same dosage can be given.

If the symptoms of asthma are clearly related to an inhaled allergen, then avoidance of that allergen is the first therapeutic step. Allergy as a cause of asthma in childhood is not common, and potentially dangerous respiratory challenges with the presumed allergen are required to prove an allergy. Hyposensitization may be helpful in some children whose asthma is due to pollens, but the mainstay of therapy is pharmacologic.

If oral theophylline in a dosage sufficient to result in good blood levels (60 to 110 μmol/L) does not relieve symptoms or produces toxic effects (irritability, hyperactivity, gastrointestinal symptoms), inhaled beta-agonists can be added to the regimen. In infants and preschool-aged children who are unable to use inhalers, the opening of a beta-agonist inhaler can be forced through the bottom of a styrofoam or paper cup, the top of the cup held over the patient's mouth and nose, and two or three puffs forced into the cup, which acts as a holding chamber (NO CLEAR EVIDENCE) (11). New spacing devices specifically designed for infants and preschool-aged children are being evaluated (12).

Because of the side effects of theophylline in some children (short attention span, restlessness, insomnia), some specialists recommend a beta-agonist inhalant as the first-choice drug, with theophylline added only if the inhaled medication by itself is insufficient. In children who have exercise-induced or cold-induced wheezing or coughing, inhaled salbutamol or cromolyn sodium, given before exercise or exposure to cold, will often prevent symptoms (FIRM EVIDENCE) (13).

If the treatments described above do not prevent or abort attacks of asthma, the child should be placed under the care of a pediatrician with training and experience in the management of moderate to severe asthma.

Croup

The care of a child with croup who is drinking well, continues to smile and play, and has no signs of respiratory distress should be managed at home. Anecdotal evidence of the efficacy of high environmental humidity has withstood the test of time. Keeping the child in the bathroom with the door and window closed and the hot water running in the shower until the room is thick with mist may alleviate symptoms. If this is not effective, having the child sit outdoors in the cool air may alleviate the cough and stridor. The value of an ordinary vaporizer for croup is unclear. If one is used, parents should be instructed that a steam vaporizer can produce severe burns if the child plays with the apparatus. Cold air vaporizers have not been shown to be more effective; although costlier, they have the advantage of safety.

If there is evidence of respiratory distress (flaring alae nasi, tachypnea, indrawing of breath, anxious expression) the child should be hospitalized and administered oxygen in an atmosphere of high humidity. Tachypnea is the best clinical predictor of the presence of hypoxemia (FIRM EVIDENCE) (14).

The efficacy of steroids in the treatment of croup is uncertain because all of the studies have major inadequacies in the design of the clinical trials (15). The efficacy of inhaled racemic epinephrine to produce short-lived improvement has led to its being used in emergency rooms, with the result that children are sent home only to be admitted later in severe distress. If racemic epinephrine is used, it should be in pediatric intensive care units by experienced personnel (16).

The care of the child who does not improve in the hospital with oxygen and humidity therapy (improvement as measured by less obvious distress, decreases in respiratory and pulse rates, and increasing arterial oxygen partial pressure) should be managed by a pediatrician in the intensive care unit. Some infants (about 2%) will require nasotracheal intubation, but even so, with appropriate care, the mortality rate is zero.

Epiglottitis

A child who is unable or unwilling to swallow and who evidences other signs of upper airway obstruction has epiglottitis, until proven otherwise. This is a true pediatric emergency. The child should be transported, while receiving oxygen, to the nearest pediatric intensive care center. Nasotracheal intubation is required. If a delay in transfer is likely to last hours, an emergency tracheostomy may be necessary if intubation is unsuccessful. The child should be accompanied in the ambulance by someone skilled in respiratory resuscitation in case this is necessary during transport to the pediatric intensive care unit.

Pneumonia

Since throat cultures do not correlate well with lung cultures (17), the choice of treatment for pneumonia in infants and children is usually based on likelihood as opposed to certitude. A blood culture in a child with pneumonia may yield a specific bacterium and thus indicate specific therapy.

In infants and preschool-aged children with pneumonia, viruses may be more common than *Streptococcus pneumoniae, Staphylococcus aureus,* or *Haemophilus influenzae* combined. Nevertheless, since it may be difficult to distinguish viral from bacterial pneumonia, amoxicillin by mouth, 40 mg/kg/day in three divided doses, can be given. If the child is too ill to take antibiotics by mouth, intravenous ampicillin, 100 mg/kg/day in four doses, is indicated. This antibiotic will cover *S. pneumoniae* and most strains of *H. influenzae.* If there is no improvement in the next 24 hours, or if the clinical condition worsens in those 24 hours, cloxacillin may be required, especially if the chest radiograph is suggestive of staphylococcal pneumonia. Cloxacillin should be administered at a dosage of 100 mg/kg/day in four divided doses. If, in spite of this therapy and attention paid to hydration and oxygenation, the child's condition does not improve, he or she should be transferred to a pediatric intensive care unit.

Chlamydial pneumonia generally responds to erythromycin, 40 mg/kg/day, or sulfisoxazole, 150 mg/kg/day (SUGGESTIVE EVIDENCE) (18). In older children with signs of pneumococcal pneumonia, oral penicillin V in doses of 50 to 100 mg/kg/day in four divided doses can be given. If the child is in a toxic condition or is unable to take oral medication, 1 or 2 days of intravenous penicillin followed by oral penicillin V should be adequate. For mycoplasmal pneumonia, erythromycin, 40 to 50 mg/kg/day, will generally shorten the course of the disease (SUGGESTIVE EVIDENCE) (19).

The parents, siblings, or caretakers (e.g., day-care workers) of any child with acute, recurrent, or chronic respiratory disease should avoid cigarette smoking (FIRM EVIDENCE) (20). Not only are children with respiratory problems adversely affected by their parents' cigarette smoking, but pulmonary function is affected in otherwise healthy children of parents who smoke.

REFERENCES

1. Glezen, W.P., Denny, F.W. Epidemiology of acute lower respiratory disease in children. *N. Engl. J. Med.* 288:498–505, 1973.

2. Pless, I.B., Roghmann, K.J. Chronic illness and its consequences: Observations based on three epidemiologic surveys. *J. Pediatr.* 79:351–359, 1971.
3. Van Dyke, R.B., Connor, J.D. Pertussis. In *Current Pediatric Therapy*, Vol. 10, Gellis, S.G., Kagan, B.M., Philadelphia: W.B. Saunders Company, 1982, p. 514.
4. Pertussis (whooping cough). In *Infectious Diseases of Children*, 8th ed. Krugman, S., Katz, S.L., Gershon, A.A., Wilfert, C., St. Louis: C.V. Mosby, 1985, p. 246.
5. Balagtas, R.C., Nelson, K.E., Levin, S., Gotoff, S.P. Treatment of pertussis with pertussis immune globulin. *J. Pediatr.* 79:203–208, 1971.
6. Altemier, W.A., III, Ayoub, E.M. Erythromycin prophylaxis for pertussis. *Pediatrics* 59:623, 1977.
7. Miller, C.L., Fletcher, W.B. Severity of notified whooping cough. *Br. Med. J.* 1:(6002)117–119, 1976.
8. Radford, M. Effect of salbutamol in infants with wheezy bronchitis. *Arch. Dis. Child.* 50:535–538, 1975.
9. Stern, R.C. Acute bronchiolitis. In Nelson, *Textbook of Pediatrics*, 12th ed., Behrman, R.E., Vaughan, V.C., eds. Philadelphia: W.B. Saunders, 1983, p. 1044.
10. Beaudry, P.H. Management of asthma in children. *Med. North Am.* 38:122–127, 1983.
11. Feldman, W. Personal communication. 1980.
12. Levinson, H., Reilly, P.A., Worsley, G.H. Spacing devices and metered-dose inhalers in childhood asthma. *J. Pediatr.* 107:662–668, 1985.
13. Gotoff, S.P. *Current Pediatric Therapy*, 10th ed. Gellis, S.S., Kagan, B.M., eds. Philadelphia: W.B. Saunders, 1982, pp. 625–626.
14. Newth, C.J.L., Levison, H., Bryan A.C. The respiratory status of children with croup. *J. Pediatr.* 81:1068–1073, 1972.
15. Tunnessan, W.W., Feinstein, A.R. The steroid-croup controversy: An analytic review of methodologic problems. *J. Pediatr.* 96:751–756, 1980.
16. Mathews, L.W. Special treatment in pediatric pulmonary disease. In *Nelson, Textbook of Pediatrics*, 12th ed., Behrman, R.E., Vaughan, V.C., eds. Philadelphia: W.B. Saunders, 1983, p. 1005.
17. Stern, R.C. The Respiratory System. In *Nelson, Textbook of Pediatrics*, 12th ed., Behrman, R.E., Vaughan, V.C., eds. Philadelphia: W.B. Saunders, 1983, p. 1051.
18. Beern, M.O., Saxon, E., Tipple, M.A. Treatment of chlamydial pneumonia of infancy. *Pediatrics* 63:198, 1979.
19. Acute Respiratory Infections. In *Infectious Diseases of Children*, Krugman, S., Katz, S.L., Gershon, A.A., Wilfert, C. Eighth edition, St. Louis: C.V. Mosby, 1985, p. 283.
20. Tager, I.B., Weiss, S.T., Rosser, B., Speizer, F.E. Effect of parental cigarette smoking on the pulmonary function of children. *Am. J. Epidemiol.* 110:15–26, 1979.

8

COMMON SKELETAL PROBLEMS

Ten to fifteen percent of all childhood injuries are skeletal, and injuries are the most common cause of morbidity and mortality in children. Failure to make a correct diagnosis or to properly treat skeletal injuries may result in permanent disability. Other skeletal problems occur as the result of abnormal growth of bones or ligaments. Aside from those caused by child abuse, skeletal injuries are rare in children less than 1 year old. Skeletal injuries are related to mobility, age, skeletal development, and the physical activities in which the child participates.

Arbitrarily, the skeletal problems discussed in this chapter are divided among the categories of sore arms, limps, and back problems. Only the most common skeletal problems are discussed; less common problems are shown in Figures 8-1 and 8-2.

PREVALENCE

The most common skeletal injury in toddlers, from when they start to walk until age 2, is fracture of the clavicle. The incidence declines between ages 2 and 6 but then rises with participation in athletics. Children aged 5 to 11 may suffer fractures of the proximal metaphysis of the humerus. Pulled elbow occurs most commonly in children aged 1 to 3 and does not occur after age 6. The so-called toddler's fracture occurs when children start walking. In children aged 10 to 13, fracture of the proximal radial head is relatively common. Less common injuries to the wrist and fingers occur in all age groups.

When infants begin walking, their parents are frequently concerned about their gait. In the first weeks of walking, 35 to 50% of children show toeing-in or -out in one or both feet. By 18 months of age, with no intervention, the incidence declines to 20%. By age 3, fewer than 1% will have persistent problems possibly requiring surgery (1).

The common causes of pain in the leg that produces a limp vary with age. In the 5- to 8-year age group, any limp or difficulty walking should be sus-

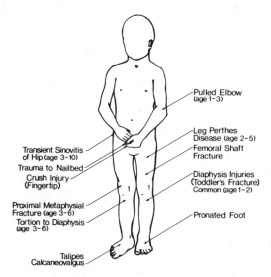

Figure 8-1. Common skeletal problems in children aged 1 to 7. (Courtesy of the Ottawa Civic Hospital.)

Figure 8-2. Common skeletal problems in children aged 8 to 18. (Courtesy of the Ottawa Civic Hospital.)

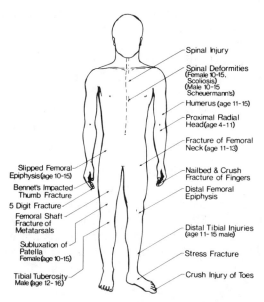

pected as being caused by Legg-Calvé-Perthes disease until proven otherwise, although it is more likely to be caused by transient synovitis of the hip. Trauma to the legs, most common in 8- to 11-year-olds, may result in fractures of the femoral shaft. Boys aged 11 to 15 are prone to fractures of the distal femoral epiphysis, usually related to trauma or sports injuries. Pain over the tibial tuberosity also occurs in approximately 2 of 1,000 adolescents. Bowlegs and knock-knee are common in newborns because of the fetal position; both remain common in toddlers until age 3. Scoliosis is primarily idiopathic and familial; it occurs eight times more frequently in pubertal girls than in boys (2).

PAINFUL OR IMMOBILE ARM

Narrowing down the problem

Clavicle fractures   Fracture of the clavicle is usually caused by a fall on the outstretched arm or a blow to the shoulder or upper chest in a fall. The fracture usually occurs in the distal or middle third of the clavicle. Simple traction, provided by a figure-of-8 bandage for 3 to 4 weeks, ensures proper healing (3).

Pulled elbow   A so-called pulled elbow is due to a tug or pull on a small child's extended arm. The radial head becomes traumatically locked from sudden traction on the hand or wrist when the elbow is extended and the forearm pronated. After such a tug, the child refuses to move the arm and holds it slightly flexed and pronated. The parents often feel guilty and upset and may believe that the arm has been paralyzed. Examination reveals tenderness over the radial head, with no restriction of flexion or extension at the elbow, but the child resists supination. Reduction is simply accomplished by flexing the elbow to 90°, placing the thumb over the radial head and then exerting mild pressure while supination of the forearm occurs. Reduction is completed with a palpable or audible click and the child can resume normal activity.

Toddler's fracture (fracture of the diaphysis of the radius and ulna)   The severity of toddler's fracture ranges from minimal green-stick deformity to complete, displaced break. The green-stick injury is manifested by angular deformities of up to 40°. Suspicion of injury should be provoked if a child has difficulty supinating or pronating the forearm, complains of pain, or has visible deformity. Once the radiological diagnosis has been made, orthopedic advice should be sought.

Fracture of the proximal radial head Fractures of the proximal radial head may be accompanied by other fractures when severe trauma is the cause. The fractures of the proximal radius are classified into three groups: mild, with less than 30° of angular deformity: moderate, with 30 to 60° of angulation; and severe, with more than 60° of angulation. Treatment usually involves im-immobilization, after correction of angulation if greater than 30°.

Fractures of the digits of the hand become more common as children become more physically active, especially in athletics. The most common injury to the thumb is Bennett's impacted fracture. If the angulation is less than 30°, straight immobilization is usually adequate treatment; however, if it is greater than 30°, the fracture should be manipulated to realign the bones before a splint and cast are applied.

Fracture of the distal radial epyphisis Because of the risk of injury to a growth center of the bone, a radiograph should be made of a wrist in which distal radial or ulnar fractures are suspected, and usually the opinion of an orthopedist should be sought. Errors in management may result in deformities and abnormal growth patterns. Fractures usually have the classical silver-fork deformity caused by dorsal displacement of the radius. Treatment requires anesthesia and involves application of direct pressure to the deformity.

Nailbed injuries Nailbed injuries tend to be neglected, but lacerations of the nailbed should be carefully sutured. Phalangeal fractures should be suspected, and, although relatively rare in children, should be managed promptly because of potential damage to the hand's future functional capability.

LIMP OR IMMOBILE LEG

Narrowing down the problem

Legg-Calvé-Perthes disease Legg-Calvé-Perthes disease usually is manifested by tenderness in the hip or pain in the hip or knee, causing a noticeable limp. Any child, especially a boy between the ages of 3 and 8, who develops these symptoms should undergo radiography of the hip to look for the characteristic flattened and fragmented femoral head with widening of the femoral neck and increase in the joint space. Reduction of weight-bearing on the joint is essential for a good outcome in adulthood. Once the disease is diagnosed, the child's condition should be assessed by an orthopedic surgeon experienced in managing the problem.

Transient synovitis   Transient synovitis of the hip is the most common cause of a painful hip in children. It affects both sexes equally between the ages of about 3 and 10 years. Transient synovitis of the hip is characterized by the sudden onset of unilateral mild to severe pain in the hip radiating to the knee and aggravated by movement or weight-bearing. Local tenderness can be palpated anteriorily over the hip joint. Motion of the hip is limited. The acute onset may be accompanied by a low-grade fever and is differentiated from Legg-Calvé-Perthes disease by the normal appearance of the joint on radiography. The inflammation is self-limited and requires no specific treatment other than rest during the acute phase, which usually lasts 5 to 10 days. Higher fever, redness or inflammation over the joint, and evidence of systemic infection suggest septic arthritis. A joint in which septic arthritis is suspected should be aspirated for diagnostic purposes and managed with the assistance of an orthopedic surgeon.

Fractured femur   A fractured femur in an infant should provoke suspicion of child abuse. Fractures of the femoral shaft are relatively common in young children and must be considered a serious injury because of the large amount of blood that is lost. The diagnosis is made on the basis of a history of a blow to the femur and marked tenderness, swelling, and immobilization of the leg, accompanied by shortening and deformity of various degrees of severity. Early, immediate management is important to reduce the amount of blood lost. When a fractured femur is suspected, a splint should be placed on the leg, and the patient carefully transported to the hospital, with minimal palpation or movement of the injured area. Assessment and management of shock are also important. Pain medication will reduce the muscle spasm around the injury and thus reduce soft tissue trauma and the risk of nerve injury.

Femoral neck fractures   Fractures of the femoral neck are most common in 11- to 13-year-olds. The diagnosis is made following severe trauma; the patient complains of severe pain in the hip and an inability to bear weight. In some cases of green-stick or impacted fracture, weight-bearing is possible. The injured limb is usually held rigid, with varying degrees of external rotation and slight abduction. There may be an actual shortening of the leg. Undisplaced fractures treated using a hip spica cast tend to heal well. There is a high risk of ischemic necrosis of the femoral head in displaced fractures and thus internal fixation is usually indicated. The treatment of these fractures should be managed by an orthopedic surgeon.

Varus or valgus deformities of the feet   It is not abnormal for a child to have considerable toeing-in or toeing-out and bowlegs during the first 3 months after starting to walk. This is usually a source of considerable anxiety for the parents and they need to be reassured. Approximately 90 to 95% of these deformities, apparent when the child first walks, resolve within 3 to 8 months.

Persistent or severe deformities may be assisted by placing medial or lateral lifts on the child's shoes, but there is NO FIRM EVIDENCE to support the use of this strategy (1). Before night splints or casts are considered, a second opinion from an orthopedic surgeon should be obtained. At large clinics, where many of these problems are handled, conservative treatment and monitoring over a 3- to 6-month period of walking have been found to be usually adequate; no specific intervention is necessary. Shoes are considered to be relatively unimportant in helping or hindering the problem as long as they fit well, are not too tight or loose, and have soft soles. A history of frequent falls or tripping that continues at least 3 months after the child has learned to walk usually signals the need for more aggressive treatment.

Femoral shaft fractures Femoral shaft fractures in 8- to 15-year-olds most commonly occur midshaft. Such fractures are serious because of the accompanying soft tissue damage and blood loss, and the potential for shock. Even with displacement, closed reduction and conservative management with immobilization is usually successful. There is good vascularization of the femoral shaft, and vascular problems are rare. Orthopedic consultation is usually required.

Fractures of the distal femoral epiphysis are usually sustained in athletic endeavors, including bicycling, skateboarding, or go-carting, or occur in injuries involving hyperextension of the knee or trauma in automobile accidents. The most common injury is hyperextension leading to anterior displacement of the epiphysis beneath the patella. The result is usually either a varus or valgus deformity associated with the variably sized metaphyseal fragments. The child complains of severe knee pain and inability to bear weight after a violent injury. The knee is often markedly swollen and tense. There may be an effusion, depending on where the fracture line is located. Because malunion leads to significant arthritic problems later in life, the treatment of these fractures should be mananged by an experienced pediatric orthopedic surgeon.

Patellar femoral knee pain Patellar subluxation usually results from a blow to the patellar region. It may mimic other injuries in the knee area as it is usually accompanied by hemorrhage, swelling, and displacement of the patella. The patella may spontaneously return to its previous location. There is evidence that a patellar dislocation is often preceded by some other type of patellar abnormality. Surgical intervention to manage these injuries is rarely indicated. Chronic subluxation is relatively common in adolescent girls and is usually associated with abnormal patella-femoral configurations or deficiencies in the supporting muscle mechanisms. Because of the lack of complete ossification of the patella, radiographic investigation is sometimes difficult or misleading. Treatment involves immobilization and a rigorous exercise program to build up the quadriceps muscles and other muscles in the knee area.

Fractures of the proximal metaphysis of the tibia and fibula Proximal metaphyseal injuries of the tibia and fibula are usually compression fractures, which heal well with closed repair and a cast. Diaphyseal injuries of the tibia result either from a direct blow or from rotational or shearing injuries. Children lack the dense bone of the adult mid- and distal third of the cortex of the tibia and are thus particularly susceptible to injuries, especially when learning to walk. The typical injury is a spiral tibial fracture, but in children between 3 and 6 years of age more torsional green-stick injuries are seen. Characteristically, the child is irritable after a fall or other incident, cries frequently, and refuses to walk or bear weight on the affected lower limb. Clinical examination often shows minimal deformity and displacement. Tenderness is localized over the distal part of the tibia. If a radiograph shows no deformity, immobilization of the bone in a cast for 3 weeks is adequate treatment.

Osgood-Schlatter disease Osgood-Schlatter disease is an inflammation of the tibial tuberosity without any fracture; it is seen more in pubertal boys than in girls. Treatment is designed to lessen the strain on the tibial tuberosity by reducing activity. Pain may necessitate the use of analgesics or nonsteroidal antiinflammatory drugs. Rarely is immobilization required. (See Chapter 22.)

Distal tibial injuries Distal tibial injuries are more common in boys, usually between the ages of 11 and 15 years. They are characterized by either rotational or triplane fractures and may present as nonspecific swelling and redness of the region. Management is sometimes difficult because of the marked swelling in the ankle region that occurs soon after the injury. Closed reduction is usually adequate, although open reduction may be necessary. The most common complication of these injuries is growth reduction in the epiphyseal plate, leading to permanent deformities of the ankle. Orthopedic advice should be obtained.

SPINAL PAIN OR DEFORMITY

Narrowing down

Spinal injury Spinal injury is very rare in prepubertal children, probably because of the flexibility of the ligaments and because the bones are not as ossified as they are in adults. It is important to note that one-half of all spinal injuries involving the spinal cord are not accompanied by a fracture.

Spinal deformities Scoliosis is the most common spinal deformity, especially in pubertal girls. Several screening methods have been proposed for the early detection of scoliosis. Unfortunately, there is NO CLEAR EVIDENCE that any method of mass screening for scoliosis has adequate sensitivity or specificity (2). The physician, in the office, should have the child bend forward from the waist after marking the spinous processes with a pen. Evidence of deviation of the spinous processes from the skin marks offers the most effective method of detecting scoliosis currently available. If there is a hump caused by the rotation of the ribs, radiographs of the spine should be made, and if there is more than a 10° angle of deviation measured by the radiologist, then an orthopedic consultation should be considered.

REFERENCES

1. Brink, K. Child foot and leg problems. *Pediatr. Ann.* 5:61, 1976.
2. Winter, R. Spine deformity in children: Current concepts of diagnosis and treatment. *Pediatrics* 5:95–112, 1976.
3. Rang, M.C. *Musculoskeletal Injuries of the Upper Limb: Care for the Injured Child.* Baltimore: Williams and Wilkins, 1975, p.10.

9

HEART MURMURS

Heart murmurs are common in children. The major goal of the physician is to differentiate the very large number of innocent murmurs from the very small number that are clinically significant. Correctly categorizing murmurs is important for two reasons: first, many parents are made anxious and the life-styles of their children restricted when an innocent murmur is said to be significant, and, second, a delay in the diagnosis of organic heart disease may result in unnecessary morbidity and, very rarely, death.

PREVALENCE

Almost 50% of children have a heart murmur (1), of which more than 99.9% are innocent if first heard after the age of 1 year. Several large surveys reveal a prevalence of congenital heart disease of 3 to 6 in 1,000 births. Of these, 86% are diagnosed by 1 year of age, almost one-half in the first week of life (2). Thus, for children one year old or older, the risk of a newly heard murmur being undiagnosed congenital heart disease is $100 - 86 = 14\% \times 6/1,000 = 0.0008$, or 8 in 10,000. Thus, fewer than 1 in 1,000 children over 1 year of age will have undiagnosed congenital heart disease. This makes it unlikely that family physicians see many children with significant heart problems in their practices. Since the experienced clinician will hear a heart murmur in 500 of 1,000 children, it is clear that insecurity on the part of the physician will lead to overdiagnosis, many unnecessary tests and referrals, and an immeasurable amount of parental anxiety. In fact, cardiac "nondisease" and the associated labeling, sick role, and limitations may be associated with more unnecessary morbidity than any other "condition" (3). Since rheumatic fever has almost disappeared in the developed world, the risk of acquired heart disease is extremely low. The annual attack rate of rheumatic fever in North America is now less than 1 per 10,000 (4).

NARROWING DOWN

The primary care physician should be concerned more with accurately separating out the innocent from the organic murmurs than with making an anatomically precise diagnosis. Some children with organic heart disease may be perfectly well at the initial assessment but be at risk of significant morbidity or early mortality later on. The lesion may not be sufficiently severe from a hemodynamic point of view to limit growth, exercise tolerance, appetite, or well-being at the time of examination, but it may predispose the child to subacute bacterial endocarditis or cardiac failure at some later date.

Table 9-1 lists the features of children who have innocent murmurs, preclinical organic murmurs, and organic heart disease. Heart disease in infants (as opposed to asymptomatic organic heart murmurs in children) will probably have been diagnosed early because of feeding or breathing problems, growth delay, or cyanosis. Such infants and children have a history of ill health, and they look and behave as if they are ill. The difficulty lies in sorting out the asymptomatic children with organic heart disease from those with innocent murmurs.

DIAGNOSIS

A positive diagnosis of an innocent heart murmur can be made on the basis of the following information:

1. Normal growth, exercise tolerance, and general health.
2. Normal skin color on physical examination.
3. No evidence of cardiac enlargement or cardiac hyperactivity.
4. Soft, vibratory, or musical grade I or II ejection systolic murmur at the left sternal border.
5. Alternatively, continuous murmur heard best at the base or right side of the neck that disappears with compression of the neck veins or when the child is supine.
6. Normally split second heart sound.
7. Normal blood pressure and femoral pulses.

Fortunately, children with innocent heart murmurs make up the vast majority of children with murmurs in a family practice. No further tests, such as electrocardiogram or chest radiograph, are necessary.

For the rare symptomatic infant, especially one who is cyanotic or having respiratory difficulty because of heart failure, the physician's suspicion of organic heart disease should be enough to stimulate an urgent consultation and probably admission to a pediatric facility.

For the asymptomatic child with a murmur that sounds organic, that is, grade 3 or more, harsh or blowing pansystolic, or diastolic, associated with a

Table 9-1. Clinical features of children with heart murmurs

Feature	Innocent murmur	Preclinical organic heart disease	Organic heart disease
Growth in relation to family's growth pattern	Appropriate	Appropriate	Short and/or thin
Exercise tolerance	Normal for age	Normal for age	Limited, mildly to severely
General health	Average number of respiratory ill-nesses for age	Average number of respiratory ill-nesses for age	Recurrent upper and lower respiratory infection; recurrent fevers; poor feeding
Inspection			
Color	Normal	Normal	Normal or cyanotic; possibly clubbing
Chest wall	Both sides of anterior chest symmetrical	Both sides of anterior chest symmetrical	If cardiomegaly, left hemithorax may bulge
Respiratory rate	Normal	Normal	May be increased
Respiratory effort	Normal	Normal	May be laboured
Palpation	Heart hits palm with a short and gentle tap	May be a thrill	May be a thrill; cardiac tap may be long and forceful
Percussion	Heart and liver not enlarged	Heart and liver not enlarged	Heart enlarged; liver enlarged if failure
Auscultation			
Loudness	Less than 3/6	1–6, usually 3 or > 3	1–6, usually 3 or > 3
Quality	Vibratory, musical	Harsh, high-pitched or blowing	Harsh, high-pitched or blowing
Location	Precordium, neck (venous hum)	Precordium, neck, back	Precordium, neck, back
Timing	Systolic ejection, diastolic (venous hum)	Systolic ejection, pansystolic, diastolic	Systolic ejection, pansystolic, diastolic
Response to neck pressure	Venous hum disappears	No change	No change
Second heart sound	Normally split	May be fixed split	May be fixed split
Blood pressure, femoral pulses	Normal, equal in arms and legs	Arm blood pressure may be high; femoral pulses absent in coarctation	Arm blood pressure may be high; femoral pulses absent in coarctation

thrill, and possibly with a fixed, split, second sound, a presumptive diagnosis of organic heart murmur can be made. A chest radiograph, electrocardiogram and echocardiogram are helpful. If ordered by the primary care physician, the films and electrocardiogram and not merely the typed report, should be made available to the consultant at the time he or she sees the patient.

For those few asymptomatic children in whom the primary care physician has difficulty distinguishing the innocent from the organic murmur, chest radiography and an electrocardiogram may be very useful. It is important, however, that whoever interprets these tests be experienced in dealing with children, so that the subtle differences between children and adults will not lead to over- or under-diagnosis.

MANAGEMENT OF HEART MURMURS

There is NO CLEAR EVIDENCE that children with innocent murmurs whose parents are told about the murmur are better (or worse) off than children whose parents are not told. In the past, when the term "heart murmur" created anxiety in and of itself, and when clinicians believed that rest was good for ill people, many parents whose children had heart murmurs (mostly innocent) limited their children's participation in competitive sports and encouraged a "sick" role. It appeared then that telling the parents about a murmur did more harm than good.

When a positive diagnosis of innocent heart murmur is made, there are theoretical reasons for mentioning it, for pointing out how prevalent such murmurs are, and for noting that a murmur is simply an extra noise in the heart or veins. If this diagnosis and its clinical insignificance are not mentioned to parents, the child may be examined by some other, less experienced clinician who may engender anxiety in the parents and order expensive tests and consultations, thereby doing more harm than good. If the parents are able to say, "We know about the murmur and have been reassured that it is innocent," such mismanagement may be prevented.

Children with organic heart disease should be monitored by a pediatric cardiologist. If there are none in the community, the question arises of who is best able to assess the condition of the child—the internist or adult cardiologist, or the general pediatrician? There is no clear answer. All pediatricians have some experience in pediatric cardiology, as part of their training. On the other hand, experience in pediatric cardiology is not mandatory in all adult-medicine training programs. Because of inexperience with children, there may be problems of over- or under-diagnosis.

The asymptomatic child with a murmur that sounds as if it could be organic but who has a normal electrocardiogram and chest radiograph should be examined at least once by a consultant to clarify the diagnosis. Only about one-third of these children will be found to have organic heart disease (5); for them, the consultant will initiate appropriate follow-up. For the other two-thirds, confirmation that the murmur is innocent will alleviate the parents', the child's, and the primary care physician's anxiety.

Children with innocent murmurs and those with preclinical organic murmurs should not be limited in their exercise. Symptomatic children will limit their own exercise. Children with organic murmurs, asymptomatic and symptomatic, should receive antibiotic prophylaxis before surgical procedures. Since subacute bacterial endocarditis is so rare, prospective controlled trials initiated to prove the efficacy of antibiotic prophylaxis would be difficult, in view of the very large sample size required. Nevertheless, since the use of prophylaxis has become established, pediatric cardiologists almost never see subacute bacterial endocarditis. If the severity of bacterial endocarditis is weighed against the minimal risks and costs of prophylaxis, prophylaxis seems the most prudent approach.

Sudden death after exertion in sports is rare in children and adolescents who have congenital heart disease; it occurs almost exclusively if aortic stenosis with a significant gradient or idiopathic hypertrophic subaortic stenosis is present. Children with these conditions may be asymptomatic but have a heart murmur that will virtually always prompt the physician to refer the child to a cardiologist. For such children, advice about participation in competitive sports should come from the consultant.

REFERENCES

1. Illingsworth R.S. *Common Symptoms of Disease in Children*, 8th ed. Oxford: Blackwell Scientific, 1984.
2. Feldt, R.H., Avasthey P., Yoshimasu, F., Kurland, L.T., Titus, J.L. Incidence of congenital heart disease in children born to residents of Olmstead County, Minnesota, 1950-1969. *Mayo Clin. Proc.* 46:794–799, 1971.
3. Morbidity of cardiac "non-disease" in school children (editorial). *Can. Med. Assoc. J.* 97:1490–1491, 1967.
4. Kempe, C.H., Silver, H.K., O'Brien, D., eds. *Current Pediatric Diagnosis and Treatment*, 8th ed. Los Altos, Calif.: Lange Medical Publications, 1984.
5. Newburger, J.W., Rosenthal, A., Williams, R.G., Fellows, K., Miettinen, O.S. Noninvasive tests in the initial evaluation of heart murmurs in children. *N. Engl. J. Med.* 308:61–64, 1983.

10

URINARY PROBLEMS

There are six main pediatric problems of the urinary system, but only two—enuresis and urinary tract infection—are relatively common. Thus, this chapter concentrates on those two problems and the other four—polyuria, abnormal urine in an asymptomatic patient, generalized edema, and hypertension—are dealt with in less detail.

PREVALENCE

Nocturnal enuresis, or involuntary nocturnal micturition that occurs at least once or twice a week, is much more common in boys than in girls. About 25% of 4-year-old and 12% of 5-year-old boys are affected. The problem declines spontaneously at a rate of about 15% per year, so that by adolescence only about 1 to 2% of boys still wet their beds (1).

Urinary tract infections may be symptomatic or asymptomatic and occur much more commonly in girls than in boys. Of the two forms of urinary tract infections, asymptomatic infections occur in about 1% of school-aged girls, and symptomatic infections occur even less often (2).

Abnormal urinalyses in asymptomatic patients, usually discovered in school-based screening programs, identify 3 to 4 in 1,000 girls and 1 in 1,000 boys who have too many red blood cells in the urine, and about 10 in 1,000 girls and 1 in 1,000 boys who have too much protein in the urine (3). High blood pressure, on the basis of statistical norms, occurs in about 3% of children; the significance of "statistical" hypertension in childhood is not clear.

Polyuria, usually associated with nocturia and polydipsia, is considered to be symptomatic of diabetes mellitus until proven otherwise. Diabetes mellitus occurs in 1 to 3 of 1,000 children less than 18 years old (4).

Generalized edema in childhood is rare and is most often caused by nephrosis, which occurs at an incidence of 2 in 100,000 children per year (5).

77

ENURESIS

Narrowing down

To identify the key clinical features that lead to the diagnosis and guide the treatment of enuresis, it is first necessary to review briefly some of the theories about causation. Since the treatments proposed depend on the concept of etiology, theories of cause and management are both summarized in Table 10-1, along with comments concerning their validity. In this discussion, primary enuresis is taken to mean nocturnal wetting in a child 5 years old or older who has never had a completely dry period lasting 6 months or more. Secondary enuresis is defined as wetting in children who have been dry for 6 months.

Diagnosis

In the child with primary enuresis who has a positive family history, no daytime symptoms, and is a deep sleeper there is most likely no serious physical or emotional cause for the problem. This is especially likely if the child is growing and developing normally and has parents who show loving concern, and for whom there is no clear-cut relationship between daytime upsets (e.g., fights with siblings, problems at school) and nighttime wetting. Good appetite and exercise tolerance virtually clinch the diagnosis. A physical examination that shows normal growth, blood pressure, tone and power in the lower extremities (the child can walk on heels, toes, hop on each leg), and a reflex tightening of the anal sphincter when the perineal skin is stroked with a cotton applicator rules out a neurological basis for the problem. Laboratory tests should be limited to routine and microscopic urinalysis and urine culture. Further investigations are unnecessary if the urine tests are negative and the child does not awaken at night to drink and has no daytime symptoms.

Management of primary enuresis

Various treatments, mainly conditioning alarms and the administration of tricyclic amines, are moderately successful and safe when used correctly. Whatever treatment is chosen, it is important to educate the child and parents that the child is not lazy, stupid, sick, or willful, and that the parents are not incompetent, cruel, or negligent. They should be told that the current theory is that this condition is a genetic sleep disorder, like sleepwalking. The basic problem is that the child sleeps too deeply to respond to the messages coming from his full bladder. A pad on the bed which triggers an alarm after a wetting episode, or a buzzer and clip-on (to underpants) electrodes may be used, especially if the child will awaken to the sound of an alarm clock. If he

Table 10-1. Proposed theories of causation and treatment of enuresis

Theory	Management based on theory	Comment on theory and management
Biomedical		
Urologic—obstruction, small bladder capacity	Intravenous pyelography, cystography, cystoscopy, urethral dilatation, bladder stretching exercises	Rarely, if ever, a cause of *nocturnal* enuresis *without* daytime dysuria, dribbling, frequency, incontinence, poor stream; radiology or cystoscopy *rarely* indicated.
Medical—diabetes mellitus, diabetes insipidus, chronic renal failure	Urinalysis, blood sugar, tests of concentrating capacity, tests of renal function	Rarely, if ever, a cause of *nocturnal* enuresis without *day* and *night* thirst and drinking, and other signs of chronic illness, e.g., fatigue, weight loss
Allergy	Elimination diets	No longer widely believed; studies purporting to show allergy as a cause seriously flawed
Psychiatric		
Freudian—penis envy, substitute masturbation, seductive mothers	Psychoanalysis of the child: treatment with alarms or pills contraindicated (will lead to symptom substitution)	Studies showing disturbances in psychosexual development seriously flawed; children successfully treated with alarms or pills show *no* symptom substitution
Disturbed family	Family therapy	Rarely a cause of *primary* enuresis; family upset usually *due to* the wetting
Psychologic, i.e., learning theory		
Proper connections between brain and bladder not learned	Conditioning apparatus, i.e., buzzer rings when bed becomes wet; reward dry nights	Moderately successful, but may not be the result of the conditioning
Genetic sleep disturbance		
Enuretic children spend more time in stage III–IV sleep, for genetic reasons	Pharmacologic management, e.g., tricyclic amines lessen amount of stage III–IV sleep, a period when wetting is likeliest; alarm system may prevent excess stage III–IV sleep	All studies show strong genetic influence, most studies show unusually deep sleep; tricyclic amine therapy moderately successful

sleeps through the noise of an alarm clock (often even when others in other bedrooms waken), it is unlikely he will awaken to the buzz of the apparatus. There is FIRM EVIDENCE that about two-thirds of children respond to buzzers and stop wetting, but the relapse rate can be high (6).

Tricyclic amines have been shown to reduce the frequency of wetting (FIRM EVIDENCE) (7), but, again, the relapse rate can be high. Occasionally, the buzzer in conjunction with the medication may work when neither is very effective alone. Some families, having been reassured that there is no medical, urologic, or psychiatric problem, prefer to wait for a remission to occur, especially if the child's self-esteem is not compromised by the wetting.

Alarms that produce an electric shock (and occasionally a first-degree burn) to the genital area may be effective (8), but constitute a form of treatment that may be worse than the problem; they should not be used.

When the diagnosis of primary enuresis is clear, referral to a specialist (urologist, nephrologist, psychologist, psychiatrist, or pediatrician with a special interest in enuresis) is not likely to be more helpful than a trial of the management already described. Some families want a second opinion; be sure the consultant will do more good than harm, that is, will not do unwarranted invasive medical, surgical, psychologic, or psychiatric investigations and therapy. Whatever program of therapy is chosen, the child and parents should chart dry and wet nights on a calendar. The child should be praised for dry nights but not punished for wet nights. Follow-up visits that focus on helping the parents enhance the child's self-esteem may be necessary for many months.

Secondary enuresis should prompt a more thorough search for stressful events, such as the arrival of a new sibling, or the start of school, or a hospitalization. Reassurance is usually enough. If the wetting persists for more than 3 months, management should be the same as for primary enuresis.

URINARY TRACT INFECTION

Narrowing down

Narrowing down the problem of urinary tract infection is not difficult in the child who presents with mainly lower tract symptoms, such as dysuria, frequency, or nocturia, with or without fever. Difficulty arises in the case of an infant under 2 years of age who cannot describe pain on urination verbally or who is still in diapers (the parents are unable to relate the crying to urination per se). Urinary tract infection should be considered in any sick-looking infant who is febrile without any discernible reason, that is, no neck stiffness or bulging fontanelle, no otitis media, no upper or lower respiratory infection, no evidence of gastroenteritis.

Occasionally, older children with pyelonephritis may have no burning on urination, but they suffer mainly abdominal or flank pain and fever. Children may have burning on urination with frequency, but without fever and with no bacteriological evidence of urinary tract infection. In this situation, chemical urethritis due to bubble bath detergent or vaginitis may be the cause.

Diagnosis

Pyuria (numerous white blood cells in the urine), often with some red blood cells present, is suggestive but does not prove infection. This may be seen in some children during the course of a nonurinary febrile illness. The absence of pyuria does not rule out infection. Bacilli seen under the microscope in an unspun urine sample is very suggestive of infection. The "gold standard" is quantitative microbiology, with 100,000 colonies per milliliter usually the accepted figure.

For infants, a bagged specimen must be sent to the laboratory very quickly, and care must be taken to avoid perineal contamination. Catheter specimens and suprapubic bladder aspirations in infants for the purpose of culture should be performed only by those experienced in collecting urine in this manner. Older children can generally cooperate in giving a midstream specimen into a sterile container. These specimens should also be processed quickly; if the laboratory is closed, the specimen should be refrigerated (not frozen) and processed as soon as the laboratory opens.

Management of urinary tract infection

In a child with dysuria, frequency, and fever—once the culture has been obtained—it is reasonable to start using antimicrobial drugs even before the laboratory results are back, especially if pyuria or bacilluria is discovered on the routine urinalysis. Trimethoprim-sulfamethoxazole (8 mg/kg trimethoprim and 40 mg/kg sulfamethoxazole per 24 hours in two divided doses) is associated with a higher initial cure rate than is sulfonamide alone, but there is a fairly high incidence of relapse whatever drug is used initially (FIRM EVIDENCE) (9). The most effective duration of initial therapy is unclear; certainly the more traditional treatment of 6 weeks has not been found to be superior to treatment for two weeks; the current debate is whether very short treatment (1 to 3 days) is as effective as 2-week treatment; different studies show different results. A conservative approach would be to treat the initial infection for 3 to 10 days. If symptoms disappear within 1 or 2 days, a follow-up culture is not necessary until 1 or 2 weeks after treatment has been concluded. Amoxicillin, 30 to 50 mg/kg/day in three divided doses, may be given instead of trimethoprim-sulfamethoxazole.

Follow-up urine cultures should be done every 3 months to attempt to identify a recurrence of infection while it is still asymptomatic; if the urine remains clear for the next year, recurrence is less likely.

For a child with recurrent symptomatic urinary tract infection (two or more attacks in 6 months), long-term trimethoprim-sulfamethoxazole therapy in half the usual daily dose given once a day is effective in preventing recurrence (FIRM EVIDENCE) (10). Depending on the frequency of recurrence, the prophylaxis should continue for 6 to 12 months, or longer if necessary. Eventually, usually within 2 years, most children outgrow the tendency toward reinfection, especially if there is no underlying structural lesion or significant persistent vesicoureteral reflux.

The child with high fever, vomiting, and abdominal or flank pain most likely has pyelonephritis, especially if there is tenderness over the costovertebral angle. Most of these children need to be hospitalized and given intravenous hydration therapy and parenteral antibiotics. Intravenous ampicillin, 100 mg/kg/24 hours in four divided doses, usually produces a prompt (within 24 hours) improvement. If there is no lessening of fever and pain in 24 hours, a resistant organism may be the cause and gentamicin, 3 mg/kg/day in three divided doses, should be given intravenously. This drug should be administered cautiously because of potential ototoxicity and nephrotoxicity; blood levels should be monitored.

In the child with clinical pyelonephritis who is not vomiting and whose parents are concerned and available to observe the results of treatment at home, a trial of oral amoxicillin, 100 mg/kg/day (dropping to 50 mg/kg/day in three divided doses once symptoms improve), can be initiated. If there is no improvement in 24 hours at home, the child should be hospitalized and intravenous therapy administered as described above.

Whereas there is still minor controversy as to which antibiotics should be given for urinary tract infection and about how long they should be given, there is much more controversy regarding the need for and timing, frequency, and type of radiologic investigation to be pursued in children with urinary tract infections. There have been no controlled trials to demonstrate that children of either sex randomly allocated to radiographic assessment after the first infection are better off than children who do not undergo assessment until the second or third episode. It is known that only about 15% of children assessed after the first episode have important structural problems, and it is in this group that recurrences are most likely. It is possible that waiting until a subsequent symptomatic or asymptomatic infection occurs will do no harm in this 15% and will obviate unnecessary irradiation of the remaining 85%.

Children with recurrent urinary tract infections who are assessed and found to have significant reflux or other radiologic abnormalities should be referred to a urologist with extensive experience in dealing with childhood urologic problems and whose approach to therapy is conservative. Such urologists are more likely to persist in a nonsurgical approach in cases in which it is not clear that surgery is necessary.

Currently, investigations into the use of renal, ureteral, and bladder ultrasound imaging are showing promising correlations with radiographic imaging. It is possible that ultrasound, which is much safer than x-irradiation, will replace intravenous pyelography and voiding cystourethrography as the procedures of choice, and that radiography will be needed only in selected cases.

If vaginitis is the cause of dysuria, a vaginal discharge is usually present. In young children, a vaginal foreign body is occasionally found. Significant discharge should be cultured for bacteria. If no organisms are cultured and symptoms persist, a wet preparation should be assessed for *Trichomonas* and a specimen sent for *candida* culture. If N. gonorrheal bacteria or *Chlamydia* are isolated, the possibility of sexual abuse must be considered in preteenagers and younger adolescents.

POLYURIA

A child who passes too much urine, is always thirsty, and wakes at night to drink as well as urinate should be suspected of having diabetes mellitus, until proven otherwise. The dipstick test for urinary glucose is the best screening test. If there is no glycosuria, the first morning urine specimen should be examined for specific gravity and osmolality. If the urine is dilute, the child may have diabetes insipidus, nephrogenic diabetes insipidus, hypercalcemia, or hypokalemia; again, referral to a pediatrician experienced in dealing with these problems is indicated. If glycosuria is found, blood glucose and electrolytes tests should be done. If hyperglycemia is present and the child is not dehydrated or vomiting, the child can be referred to a consultant within the next day or so. If there is vomiting and dehydration, an intravenous infusion of normal saline should be started, with 30 mEq/L of potassium added when the child voids. The formula for maintenance fluids (see Chapter 27) can be used and supplemented with an additional 50 ml/kg/24 hours. Urgent referral to a consultant is indicated.

ABNORMAL URINALYSIS IN AN ASYMPTOMATIC CHILD

Proteinuria

If there are no red blood cells or casts in the urine and the child is well, the child should be tested for orthostatic proteinuria: the child should empty his or her bladder at bedtime and be awakened again to void in the toilet before the parents retire. He or she should then remain in bed, recumbent, until awakening next morning and then should void into a marked bottle before getting out of bed. This specimen should be labeled "A.M. specimen." The child should then engage in normal activity until approximately 4 P.M., when he or she should void into a bottle labeled "4 P.M. specimen." The two specimens should be checked for protein using a dipstick. If there is no or a trace of protein in the A.M. specimen and more in the P.M. specimen, then the child has orthostatic proteinuria, a benign condition that requires no further investigation. If both specimens contain more than 30 milligrams of protein, the child should be referred to a pediatric consultant. Although many children with nonorthostatic proteinuria do not have significant pathology, treatable renal conditions that result in chronic renal failure may occasionally be manifested in this way.

Hematuria

Most healthy children whose urine shows blood by dipstick or microscopy do not have serious pathology; some may have benign, recurrent, gross hematuria without significant renal histopathology. Nevertheless, there are some sinister, treatable conditions, such as systemic lupus erythematosus, that may begin with asymptomatic gross or microscopic hematuria; thus, children with this finding should be referred to a pediatric consultant.

Because so few children with significant, treatable renal diseases are identified by mass urinary screening programs in the schools, and because it is not known how many of them would soon be symptomatic and therefore report to their physicians for treatment, most authorities do not recommend mass screening of children for urine abnormalities. Routine urinalysis in office practice is also not indicated for healthy children during well-child examinations.

GENERALIZED EDEMA

Children with edema (puffy eyelids, ascites, leg edema) should be assumed to have nephrotic syndrome until proven otherwise. Occasionally, children with acute post-streptococcal glomerulonephritis have the same symptoms, but gross hematuria is the usual key feature in that disease. Children with bilaterally swollen eyelids that are not inflamed should have a urine dipstick test done for protein and blood. If there is heavy proteinuria and no or trace blood in the urine, and the child is otherwise well (no hypertension, no dyspnea), he or she probably has a benign form of childhood nephrosis. Nevertheless, because relatively high doses of steroids are required for treatment and attention must be paid to blood volume and electrolytes, the help of a pediatric consultant is recommended.

HYPERTENSION

A child who is symptomatic (gross hematuria, headache, dyspnea) and hypertensive represents a pediatric emergency and should be referred to a hospital immediately. Such children usually have acute glomerulonephritis.

Although this condition has an excellent prognosis, seizures and heart failure may occur within the first few days. Most children who are hypertensive are asymptomatic and are usually identified in their physician's office during routine health check-ups. Repeated measurements, using the proper size cuff, that show a diastolic blood pressure above 75 mm Hg in a prepubertal child and above 85 mm Hg in an adolescent represent a statistical (greater than ninety-fifth percentile) abnormality and possibly a long-term clinical problem as well. Controversy exists as to how vigorous the investigation should be for the cause of the hypertension and how aggresive the treatment should be, since the long-term natural history of asymptomatic hypertension is unknown. A reasonable approach has been suggested by the U.S. Task Force on Blood Pressure Control in Children (11):

1. Obtain the family's history of hypertension and its complications.
2. Record blood pressure of parents and siblings.
3. Review patient's history for evidence of renal disease or drugs that may elevate the pressure.
4. Perform a physical examination: record blood pressure in all four limbs; perform funduscopy; assess heart size; look for femoral pulses, café au lait spots (neurofibromatosis can be associated with hypertension); listen for flank bruits; look for evidence of hyperthyroidism.
5. Determine blood urea nitrogen level as well as creatinine and perform routine urinalysis: if all are normal, further tests are unnecessary.
6. Recommend a weight reduction program if the child is obese.
7. Recommend that the child avoid excessive salt (more than 8 g NaCl/day) in the diet.
8. Encourage a dynamic exercise program.
9. Discourage smoking.

If this approach is not successful in lowering the blood pressure and if the recordings are consistently above 130/80 in a prepubertal child or 140/90 in an adolescent, the patient should be referred to a pediatric consultant.

REFERENCES

1. Feldman, W. Enuresis. In *Advances in Behavioural Medicine for Children and Adolescents*, Firestone, P., McGrath, P.J., Feldman, W., eds. Hillsdale, N.J: Lawrence Erlbaum Associates, 1983, p. 104.
2. Kunin, C.M. Epidemiology and natural history of urinary tract infection in school age children. *Pediatr. Clin. North Am.* 18:509–528, 1971.
3. West, C.D. Asymptomatic hematuria and proteinuria in children: Causes and appropriate diagnostic studies. *J. Pediatr.* 89:173–182, 1976.
4. O'Brien, D. Diabetes mellitus. In *Current Pediatric Diagnosis and Treatment*, 8th ed., Kempe, C.H., Silver, H.K., O'Brien, D., eds. Los Altos, Calif.: Lange Medical Publications, 1984, p. 786.

5. Chan, J.C.M. Urinary tract diseases. In *Pediatrics*, H.M. Maurer, ed. New York: Churchill Livingstone, 1983, p. 476.
6. Doleys, D.M. Behavioral treatments for nocturnal enuresis in children: A review of the recent literature. *Psychol. Bull.* 84:30–54, 1977.
7. Kolvin, I., Taunch, J. Currah, J., Garside, R.F., Nolan, J., Shaw, W.B. Enuresis: A descriptive analysis and a controlled trial. *Dev. Med. Child Neurol.* 14:715–726, 1972.
8. McKendry, J.B., Stewart, U.A., Khanna, F., Netley, C. Primary enuresis: Relative success of three methods of treatment. *Can. Med. Assoc, J.* 113:953–955, 1975.
9. Feldman, W., Johnson, D.M., Newberry, P., Weldon, A., Naidoo, S. Comparison of trimethoprim-sulfamethoxazole with sulfamethoxazole in urinary tract infections of children. *Can. Med. Assoc. J.* 112:195–215, 1975.
10. Smellie, J.M., Katz, G., Gruneberg, R.N. Controlled trial of prophylactic treatment in childhood urinary-tract infection. *Lancet* 2:175–178, 1978.
11. Recommendations of the task force on blood pressure control in children. *Pediatrics* 59 (suppl.):797–810, 1977.

11
FITS AND FAINTS

Fits and faints are episodic or paroxysmal alterations in consciousness. They are manifested clinically as apneic spells (especially in infancy), breath-holding attacks, febrile seizures, recurrent afebrile seizures (epilepsy), and vasovagal syncope, orthostatic hypotension, and hyperventilation syndrome. The last three entities are more common in adolescents.

PREVALENCE

Apneic spells in infancy are uncommon. The condition is defined as apnea lasting longer than 15 seconds, followed either by spontaneous resumption of breathing or resuscitation. Exact prevalence figures are unknown, but a children's hospital serving an area whose population is greater than 1,000,000 handled only twenty-eight cases in 2 years (1).

Breath-holding attacks, defined as apneic episodes following anger, frustration, or pain, occur in about 5% of preschool-aged children.

Febrile seizures, simple or complex, occur in about 3% of children between the ages of 6 months and 6 years (2). Simple febrile seizures occur in children in this age group and are characterized by generalized seizures lasting 15 minutes or less in neurologically and developmentally normal children who have no focal neurological signs and who have either high or rapidly rising body temperature. Complex febrile seizures are seizures accompanied by fever that are in any way different from simple febrile seizures. Fortunately, most children who suffer from febrile seizures have the simple form.

Recurrent afebrile seizures, or epilepsy, occur in fewer than 1% of children (3).

Vasovagal syncope, or fainting, usually occurs when a child is frightened (e.g., after hypodermic injection) and is caused by a sudden drop in blood pressure when the child is in the upright position. The exact prevalence is unknown, but such fainting is not rare.

Orthostatic hypotension, or a feeling of lightheadedness or of fainting, occurs mainly in adolescents when they rise suddenly from a lying or sitting position. The prevalence is unknown, but the condition is felt to be fairly common.

Some teenagers, more often girls, experience lightheadedness or "blackouts" when they are anxious, the result of hyperventilation and the associated hypocapnea and respiratory alkalosis. The prevalence of this hyperventilation syndrome is unknown, but it is not rare.

APNEIC SPELLS

Narrowing down

An infant in an apneic spell appears lifeless to the caretaker, which often prompts attempts at resuscitation. About 50% of these babies have no demonstrable cause for the sudden cessation of breathing; the others have either gastroesophageal reflux with aspiration of gastric contents, or an underlying central nervous system disorder, such as epilepsy (1). This infant apnea syndrome is referred to by other terms, for example, near-miss sudden infant death syndrome.

Diagnosis

Because some infants with the infant apnea syndrome will ultimately die of sudden infant death syndrome, and because some have treatable causes of apnea (gastroesophageal reflux, epilepsy), they should be referred to a pediatric center where there are consultants experienced in dealing with such infants. They will most often undergo a period of respiratory monitoring, electroencephalograms, metabolic studies, and possibly an esophageal pH probe study.

Management of apneic spells

If the cause of the apneic spells can be identified (in fewer than 50% of cases is the cause identifiable), then the treatment is that of the underlying cause, for instance, of gastroesophageal reflux or seizure disorder. In other cases, theophylline, which has a respiratory stimulating effect, has been used, but its use has not been eveluted in older infants in randomized controlled trials. The use of a home apnea monitor is widely recommended; to date, there have been no randomized controlled clinical trials designed to determine whether home apnea monitors (a) save lives or (b) diminish or increase parental anxiety. If an apnea monitor is to be used in the home, instruction in its use and in resuscitation should be provided by an experienced team. False alarms generate great anxiety and may lead to a "cry wolf" situation. Similarly, if the alarm is sounded because of real apnea and the parents have no knowledge of basic resuscitation techniques, the child may die in front of his or her help-less, frustrated, anguished parents. The mainstay of treatment is reassur-ance—most infants with the infant apnea syndrome do not progress to sudden infant death syndrome (1), whether or not there is home apnea monitoring.

BREATH-HOLDING ATTACKS

Narrowing down

The main condition to consider in addition to simple breath-holding—espe-cially if the episode is followed by loss of consciousness or a seizure—is epilepsy. Breath-holding occurs in children between the ages of 6 months and 5 years and peaks at around 12 to 18 months. The child, when frustrated or in pain, will cry, maintain a respiratory position of expiration, and not in-spire again until all the adults around him have been thoroughly frightened. Generally, this prolonged expiratory phase is not consciously maintained and is not, at least initially, performed in an attempt to manipulate the caretakers. Most children, when in pain or thwarted, will cry but will inspire before they lose consciousness; some children will have an anoxic loss of con-sciousness, with or without a generalized seizure, before they commence regular breathing.

Diagnosis

If the physician has the opportunity to observe one of these episodes, the diagnosis is quite easy: there is no other condition that causes an angry or pained child to maintain a position of expiration, almost invariably following crying, that leads to cyanosis or pallor, often a loss of consciousness, and, rarely, a short-lived, generalized seizure. The results of the physical examina-tion will be normal, and the key feature in the history will be that these episodes always follow some stressful or painful event. If the attack occurs without apparent provocation or crying, investigations, including an elec-troencephalogram, may be necessary; in almost all cases, the history is diag-nostic.

Management of breath-holding attacks

The treatment of breath-holding consists of educating the parents that (a) breath-holding spells are not caused by and do not cause brain damage, (b) all infants and children outgrow these episodes eventually, (c) most infants and children with this condition learn that crying not only compels attention but, in most families, will get them anything they want. Parents reinforce the crying behavior by catering to the child's every whim, in fear that a bout of crying will lead to breath-holding. It is, therefore, very important to teach parents that breath-holders should be treated like any other infant or child. That is, reasonable requests for attention, candy, television, or whatever should be met, but unreasonable requests should not be, even if it is clear that thwarting will lead to breath-holding. In virtually all breath-holders treated consistently in this manner, the frequency and severity of breath-holding will decrease; conversely, rewarding the crying behavior will lead to progressive increases in the child's manipulative behavior. It is important to have both parents present for this discussion and to assess whether both can comply. Follow-up is required.

FEBRILE SEIZURES

Narrowing down

Febrile seizures must be differentiated from meningitis, either bacterial or viral, which can also be manifested by fever and a seizure in the 6-month to 6-year-old age group. As well, epilepsy or other neurological conditions can be manifested as a fit when the seizure threshold is lowered because of fever. Hypocalcemic seizures, usually due to rickets, have to be considered in cow's milk–fed infants born in the fall and on a farm, and who drink milk that does not contain added vitamin D. In addition, infants of breast-feeding vegan vegetarian mothers who do not receive adequate sunlight are at risk of developing rickets and hypocalcemic fits, which may be coincidental with a febrile illness.

Diagnosis

The major question to be asked when confronted with what appears to be a febrile seizure is, should a lumbar puncture be performed or not? Since life-threatening meningitis can result in fever and a convulsion, what has to be done to rule out meningitis? Many pediatric centers recommend lumbar punctures for all children who have experienced a convulsion. There are several reasons for questioning this recommendation:

1. In infants more than 6 months old, meningeal signs (stiff neck, Kernig's sign, Brudzinski's sign, bulging fontanelle) are present by the time the seizure occurs in a considerable majority of cases of meningitis. Certainly, when there is any suspicion of meningitis, the child should undergo a lumbar puncture.
2. The seizure itself in meningitis is often different from that of a simple febrile seizure; it may be focal, last more than 15 minutes, or be as-

sociated with postictal focal signs. Such children should undergo a lumbar puncture.

3. Following the seizure, and even after antipyretic measures have been taken, a child with meningitis will still look very sick: the child may not make eye contact, not respond to his or her parents, and be unconsolable and either irritable or lethargic. On the other hand, a child who has had a simple febrile seizure, will, usually 1 hour after antipyretic measures have been taken, be very alert, may even be playful, and will maintain eye contact; the parents will almost always state that the child appears normal again.

4. Lumbar puncture is very painful.

5. A lumbar puncture may convert a fairly common, usually benign, cause of fever—pneumococcal bacteremia—into meningitis if the needle breaks down the blood-brain barrier (4).

6. Using a policy of selective lumbar punctures in children with fever and seizures, we at the Children's Hospital of Eastern Ontario performed lumbar punctures in only one-third of such patients and missed no cases of meningitis. Thus, two-thirds of patients safely avoided the procedure.

Thus a child with a typical, simple febrile seizure, who is alert and responsive once the fever has decreased and who can be observed in an emergency room setting for several hours to ensure normal central nervous system functioning, does not need to undergo a lumbar puncture. In an infant under 6 months of age in whom meningeal signs may not be so obvious, and in an older infant in whom there are any questions remaining after the history or physical examination, a lumbar puncture should be done.

The cause of the fever leading to the febrile seizure should also be investigated. If there is no obvious cause (otitis media, upper respiratory infection, pneumonia, gastroenteritis), a urinalysis and urine culture are reasonable and inexpensive tests. The sensitivity, specificity, and predictive value of other tests (blood culture, complete blood cell count, erythrocyte sedimentation rate) are not sufficiently helpful to make their use routine in these circumstances.

In the typical case of febrile seizures, electroencephalography is not helpful. The EEG is usually normal several weeks after the seizure. Even if there are abnormalities, the management of the care of the child with regard to anticonvulsants and follow-up is based much more on clinical findings than on any EEG changes.

Management of febrile seizures

Children with simple febrile seizures have an excellent prognosis. The risk of epilepsy developing in this group of children is only marginally greater than that in children who have never had febrile seizures (11 per 1,000 versus 5 per 1,000)(2). How this is presented to the parents is very important. If one says that the child has twice the risk of developing epilepsy, a great deal of anxiety may be engendered. On the other hand, parents are likely to be much less anxious (and to treat their child in a less overprotected manner) if they are told that the chances that their child will not develop epilepsy are about 99 to 1 and that the prophylactic administration of anticonvulsant drugs for simple febrile seizures is not indicated. Phenobarbital prophylaxis has been shown to prevent subsequent febrile seizures (FIRM EVIDENCE) (5), and since 30 to 40% of children will experience recurrences, it would seem at first glance that prophylaxis makes sense. However, it is clear that even recurrent simple febrile seizures are associated with an excellent prognosis, whereas the risk of significant long-term behavioral and cognitive side effects of daily anticonvulsants over 2 or more years may be greater than the benefit. The recommendations of Camfield et al. (5) to restrict prophylaxis to patients with complex febrile seizures or to children who live in remote areas who have limited access to medical care seem reasonable.

EPILEPSY

Narrowing down

A history of recurrent afebrile seizures is in fact the definition of epilepsy; narrowing down in this context is done merely in the effort to find a cause for the disorder. Space-occupying lesions, such as brain tumors or subdural hemotomas, or metabolic conditions associated with hypoglycemia or hypocalcemia, are the major problems to pursue because they are treatable, though rare. One form of epilepsy that may present diagnostic problems is complex partial seizures, previously termed psychomotor epilepsy. This condition is characterized by alterations in consciousness, unresponsiveness, visual distortions, and feelings of intense fear. Patients may resist restraint or react angrily to objects or persons in their way. The key point in the history is that the child behaves in a totally uncharacteristic way with no provocation.

Diagnosis

An electroencephalogram is probably the single most important laboratory test in evaluating a child suspected of having epilepsy. A normal EEG does not rule out epilepsy. In cases in which the family doctor is uncertain, a referral is indicated. Some pediatric neurologists regularly perform a lumbar puncture in any infant seen at the time of the first seizure, whether or not the infant is febrile (6). There is NO CLEAR EVIDENCE that routine lumbar puncture is needed. Computerized tomographic (CAT) scanning is best ordered by a physician experienced in dealing with large numbers of epileptic children. In one study, only 3 in 1,000 children who had been having seizures for 3 years and who had no central nervous system signs were found to have a brain tumor (6). Other tests, such as metabolic screening tests, should be performed on a selective basis.

Management of epilepsy

The medical management of epilepsy is generally not complicated. In many cases, a single anticonvulsant drug, in appropriate doses, will abolish or markedly decrease the seizures without producing significant side effects. Whether the family doctor or a specialist manages a patient's seizure disorder depends on a variety of factors: the experience of the primary care physician in diagnosing and treating epilepsy, pressures from the family for referral, and the availability and accessibility of either a general pediatric consultant with experience in treating epilepsy or a pediatric neurologist. Most primary care physicians prefer to refer epileptic children to a consultant because the management of the care of such children, which includes education as well as compliance-enhancing strategies, is time-consuming and requires knowledge of the rapidly developing field of anticonvulsive pharmacology. Although referral to a pediatric neurologist has been recommended even when the physician suspects syncope or breath-holding (7), there is NO CLEAR EVIDENCE that such a referral is necessary if the diagnosis of either of these conditions is clear.

Whichever physician is responsible for choosing and monitoring anticonvulsant therapy (see standard pediatric texts for drugs and dosages), the child and family, and occasionally the child's teachers, must also be educated about the disorder. The primary care physician should ensure that this education is carried out. The parents must learn that their child is not an epileptic—their child is a child who is prone to seizures. As for all childhood chronic diseases, the emphasis should not be on disease but on health. The child with epilepsy should have the same rights and responsibilities, rewards and privileges, as other children. Educators and parents must learn how to deal with seizures, especially that they should not put objects in the child's mouth, panic, or create a scene. In most cases, the seizure will resolve spontaneously; if not, the child should be taken to the hospital. The child and family should also be made aware that the prognosis for the majority of children with epilepsy is very good. Even if a consultant has been involved at the beginning, many family physicians do an excellent job of monitoring the child's condition, especially once seizures are controlled. There is NO CLEAR EVIDENCE that routine anticonvulsant blood level determinations are necessary for a child whose seizures are controlled without side effects.

VASOVAGAL SYNCOPE, ORTHOSTATIC HYPOTENSION, HYPERVENTILATION

Narrowing down

Syncope has to be differentiated from epilepsy, either true or hysterical. The prodrome of the faint consists of feelings of weakness, warmth, and nausea, and blurring of vision. This prodrome occurs following the stimulus (sight of blood, hypodermic injection, standing in the heat) and is different enough from that in epilepsy to distinguish the two conditions. The premonitory symptoms are valuable, especially if there are brief convulsive movements following the fainting episode.

Orthostatic hypotension is virtually always distinguishable from vasovagal syncope, epilepsy, and hyperventilation because it alone occurs with a sudden change in position, from lying or sitting to standing.

Teenagers with hyperventilation syndrome feel lightheaded but rarely lose consciousness, which thereby distinguishes this syndrome from syncope and epilepsy. The patients almost always complain of numbness and tingling in the extremities. The symptoms are caused by hypocapnia, alkalosis, and decreased cerebral blood flow. They are not relieved by lying down. Although the patient may not be aware of it, other observers note that his or her pattern of breathing is abnormal during the episode.

Diagnosis

For syncope, orthostatic hypotension, and hyperventilation, laboratory tests are rarely necessary. The characteristic history of each and the normal results of the physical examination in all three should allow the clinician to be secure in the diagnosis. In the hyperventilation syndrome, having the adolescent abort an attack by breathing into a paper bag will not only convince the clinician of the diagnosis but also the child and the family. In this instance, successful therapy confirms the diagnosis.

Management of syncope, orthostatic hypotension, and hyperventilation

Vasovagal syncope If the stimuli that provoke fainting are known (blood-taking, hypodermic injection) and they are unavoidable, the particular procedure should be done when the child is lying down. After the procedure, the child should stay in that position, and arise slowly. Standing at attention for prolonged periods in a stuffy room should be avoided; at the first premonitory symptoms, the child should leave the room and lie down. The physiological mechanism—reflex slowing of the heart and hypotension leading to transient brain hypoxia—and the benign nature of these episodes should be thoroughly explained to child and family. Teachers should also understand the benign nature of "fainting," as well as how to prevent it and how to alleviate anxiety in the child and his or her peers when an episode occurs.

Orthostatic hypotension The physiology of the condition—peripheral vasodilatation and pooling of blood in the legs leading to transient brain hypoxia—should be explained to the child and the family. Adolescents should be instructed never to stand quickly from a lying or sitting position. The benign nature of these episodes should be emphasized.

Hyperventilation syndrome The physiology of the syndrome should be explained, and the relief of symptoms secondary to rebreathing carbon dioxide should be demonstrated. The teenager should be prepared to use a paper bag if symptoms develop. If the attacks are frequent and socially incapacitating, or if there is other evidence of psychosocial dysfunction, then the individual and family should be assessed by the primary care physician, if he or she is interested and skilled, or by a consultant. Relaxation techniques or other behavior management strategies can be tried (NO CLEAR EVIDENCE of efficacy).

REFERENCES

1. Camfield, P., Camfield, C., Bagnell, P., Rees, E. Infant apnea syndrome. *Clin. Pediatr.* 21:684–687, 1982.
2. Nelson, K.B., Ellenberg, J.H. Predictors of epilepsy in children who have experienced febrile seizures. *N. Engl. J. Med.* 295:1029–1033, 1976.
3. Chutorian, A.M. Paroxysmal disorders of childhood. In *Pediatrics*, Rudolph A.M., and Hoffman, J.I.E., eds. Norwalk, Conn.: Appleton-Century-Crofts, 1982, p. 1871.
4. Teele, D.W., Daskofsky, B., Rakusan, T., Klein, J.O. Meningitis after lumbar puncture in children with bacteremia. *N. Engl. J. Med.* 305:1079–1081, 1981.
5. Camfield, P.R., Camfield, C.S., Shapiro, S.H., Cummings, C. The first febrile seizure—antipyretic instruction plus either phenobarbital or placebo to prevent recurrence. *J. Pediatr.* 97:16–21, 1980.
6. Pedley, T.A., DeVivo, D.C. Seizure disorders in infants and children. In *Pediatrics*, Rudolph A.M., and Hoffman, J.I.E., eds. Norwalk, Conn.: Appleton-Century-Crofts, 1982, p. 1665.
7. Leicher, C. Seizures in infancy and childhood. In *Primary Care Pediatrics, a Symptomatic Approach*, Shelov, S.P., Mezey, A.P., Edelmann, C.M., and Barnett, H.L., eds. Norwalk, Conn.: Appleton-Century-Crofts, 1984, p. 228.

12

LUMPS AND BUMPS

This chapter deals with visible or palpable masses in children. Excluded are skin problems, which are discussed in Chapter 6. The chapter is divided into two sections, the first covering the visible anomalies found at birth (see Fig. 12-1), the second covering lumps and bumps that appear after the age of approximately 1 month (see Fig. 12-2). The two sections are subdivided by the physical locations of the lumps. The text deals with the most common abnormalities; more detail is shown in the figures and in Table 12-1. Injuries, probably the most common cause of lumps or bumps in children, are discussed in Chapter 24.

NEWBORN TO 1 MONTH

Head and face

Dermoid cysts Dermoid cysts occur on the skull wherever two cranial bones join. Most commonly, dermoid cysts are seen unilaterally under the eyebrow or on the outer edge of the eyebrow. They also may occur in the midline or on the parietal suture. The cysts can be superficial to the bone or part of the bone, making the differential diagnosis of these cysts from simple intradermal cysts difficult. That a cyst occurs in a newborn is most suggestive of a dermoid cyst. A surgical consultant will confirm the diagnosis; dermoid cysts can usually be removed without difficulty.

Periauricular sinuses Embryological defects produced by faulty closure around the external ear result in periauricular sinuses, cysts, or tags. Rarely do sinuses produce any significant problems. Surgical intervention may be considered for cosmetic reasons.

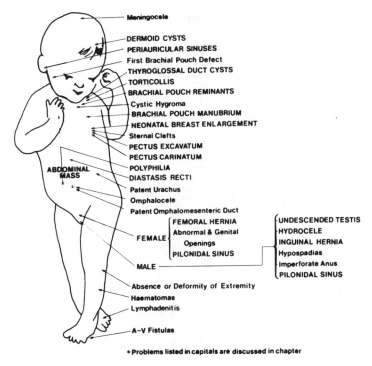

Figure 12-1. Lumps and bumps in newborns and infants. (Courtesy of the Ottawa Civic Hospital.)

Neck

Thyroglossal duct cyst Any lesion in the neck close to the midline should be considered a possible thyroglossal duct cyst. Thyroglossal duct cysts usually occur between the hyoid bone and the manubrium sterni, most commonly within 2 or 3 centimeters of the hyoid bone. They can be present at birth or may appear fairly suddenly later on. Thyroglossal duct cysts should be removed by a surgical consultant because they tend to become infected.

Torticollis Congenital torticollis is usually secondary to shortening of the sternocleidomastoid muscle and is probably caused by tearing of the muscle in utero due to excessive fetal activity. The muscles heal by fibrosis and contracture, leaving a shortened muscle. Clinically, torticollis is difficult to diagnose unless the clinician moves the child's head laterally to the right and left. The muscle segment where fibrous healing occurs often becomes a visible or palpable mass. With early diagnosis, torticollis is most easily treated by ap-

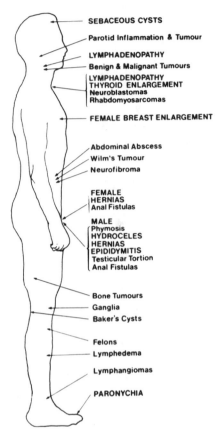

SEBACEOUS CYSTS

Parotid Inflammation & Tumour

LYMPHADENOPATHY

Benign & Malignant Tumours

LYMPHADENOPATHY
THYROID ENLARGEMENT
Neuroblastomas
Rhabdomyosarcomas

FEMALE BREAST ENLARGEMENT

Abdominal Abscess

Wilm's Tumour

Neurofibroma

FEMALE
HERNIAS
Anal Fistulas

MALE
Phymosis
HYDROCELES
HERNIAS
EPIDIDYMITIS
Testicular Tortion
Anal Fistulas

Bone Tumours

Ganglia

Baker's Cysts

Felons

Lymphedema

Lymphangiomas

PARONYCHIA

Figure 12-2. Lumps and bumps in children aged 1 month to 15 years. (Courtesy of the Ottawa Civic Hospital.)

propriate exercises to stretch the sternocleidomastoid muscle. If the condition is not diagnosed before 3 or 4 months of age, or if exercises are not satisfactory, then surgical incision of the muscle may be necessary. If the problem is diagnosed much later than 4 to 6 months, opthalmologic problems may develop since the child sees the world at a tilt.

Thorax

Brachial pouch defect of the manubrium Brachial pouch defects can be found on the manubrium of the thorax. They often appear as one or two tiny sinus tracts that produce a salivalike fluid. They may be removed for cosmetic reasons.

Table 12-1. Lumps and bumps in children

	Head and face	Neck	Thorax	Abdomen	Ano-genital region Male	Ano-genital region Female	Extremities
Newborns and infants	Dermoid cyst Periauricular sinus First brachial pouch defect	Thyroglossal duct cyst Torticollis Brachial pouch Cystic hygroma	Brachial pouch defect of the manubrium Neonatal breast enlargement Sternal cleft Pectus excavatum Pectus carinatum Polyphilia	Patent urachus Omphalocele Patent omphalomesenteric duct	Undescended testis Hydrocele Inguinal hernia Hypospadias Imperforate anus	Femoral hernia Abnormal anogenital openings Pilonidal sinus	Absence or deformity Hamartoma Lymphadenitis Arteriovenous fistula
Children more than 2 months old	Lymphadenopathy Sebaceous cyst Parotid inflammation and tumor Benign and malignant tumor	Lymphadenopathy Thyroid enlargement Neuroblastoma Rhabdomyosarcoma	Precocious breast enlargement Gynecomastia in pubertal males	Abdominal abscess Wilms' tumor Neurofibroma Polycystic kidney	Phymosis Hydrocele Hernia Epididymitis Testicular torsion Anal fistula	Hernia Anal fistula Pieinoidal sinus	Ganglia Baker's cyst Paronychia Lymphedema Lymphangioma

Neonatal breast engorgement The most common abnormality in the exterior thoracic region is the enlargement of the breasts in both males and females in the neonatal period. It is due to stimulation of the breast tissue by maternal estrogen and it normally subsides within 4 to 6 weeks. It may be extensive enough to produce masses in the breast tissue, but abscesses rarely occur. Other than the reassurance of the parents, no further treatment is necessary.

Pectus excavatum Pectus excavatum may occur from birth through age 4 to 6 years. It is primarily a cosmetic problem. Repair of severe pectus excavatum may be justified in a child over the age of 6 if the cosmetic defect interferes with the development of the child's self-esteem.

Pectus carinatum Pectus carinatum, also known as pigeon breast, is caused by more rapid growth of the ribs than of the rest of the thoracic bone structure. No physiological defect has been associated with pectus carinatum, and therefore surgical repair is done for cosmetic reasons only. A mixed defect of both carinatum and excavatum also may occur, but unless the pectus excavatum is severe, the defect has no physiological implication.

Polyphilia—Supernumerary breast It is not uncommon for extra breast tissue to develop unilaterally or bilaterally, extending from the axilla down to the lower abdominal area. These supernumerary nipples lie in the vertical line of the normal nipple. Surgical intervention should be considered only for cosmetic reasons.

Abdomen

Diastasis recti Occasionally, the connection between the two rectus muscles in the abdomen is absent. This is not an abnormality but only a variation of normal anatomy; reassurance of the parents is important.

Umbilical hernia Umbilical hernias are extremely common in children and, unless they become incarcerated, will normally close spontaneously. Surgical intervention for an umbilical hernia should not be made until the child is at least 5 years old, by which time virtually all hernias will have disappeared. The main problem is convincing worried parents of this. Umbilical hernias are more common in children with congenital hypothyroidism.

Genitals—Male

Undescended testis An undescended testis may appear anywhere along the area between the anterior superior iliac spine and the pubic tubercle. It occurs in 3% of full-term males, 20% of prematures males, and up to 70% of babies weighing less than 1,500 grams at birth. Two-thirds of all undescended testicles will descend within the first year (1, 2). If, after compression along this line, a testicle is not felt, there probably is an undescended testicle. Approximately 90% of undescended testicles are accompanied by an indirect inguinal hernia. An undescended testicle should be surgically repaired prior to the age of 2 years because of subsequent marked decline in spermatogenesis. With untreated cryptorchidism, men have a much greater incidence of testicular cancer (2, 3). There is NO CLEAR EVIDENCE that nonspontaneous testicular descent will respond to treatment with human chronic gonadotropin (4).

Hydrocele   A hydrocele is a collection of fluid at the bottom of a hernial sac. Physiological hydroceles that are present at birth will often disappear within 3 months. Hydroceles are considered significant only after the age of 4 months, when they usually indicate an inguinal hernia. If the size fluctuates after 4 months, this is further evidence of a hernia rather than of a hydrocele and indicates the need for surgical repair.

Inguinal hernia   Direct inguinal hernias are rare in children. Indirect inguinal hernias are most often detected by the palpation of a tightening of the spermatic cord on one side. The normal method of examining an adult—having the patient increase the intraabdominal pressure so the physician can feel the enlargement of the inguinal hernia—is contraindicated and misleading in infants. The main complication of an inguinal hernia is incarceration. Thus, if a hernia is suspected in an infant, a consultation is indicated. A child with an incarcerated inguinal hernia has acute abdominal pain and shows signs of bowel obstruction. Palpation of the hernial area will not reveal a mass but will usually detect tenderness.

Pilonidal sinus   Pilonidal sinuses can be seen at birth but rarely become infected in children. If one does, it should be treated by incision and drainage. There is NO CLEAR EVIDENCE that prophylactic removal is necessary.

Genital—Female

There are no commonly found masses in the female genital region.

Extremities

There are no commonly found masses in the extremities of a newborn.

1 MONTH TO 18 YEARS

Head and face

Lymphadenopathy   Palpable lymph nodes are common in the suboccipital region: they are usually the result of scalp lesions, scratches caused by a comb, or minor trauma. These lymph nodes should be differentiated from sebaceous cysts or dermoid cysts, which may also occur in this region. The nodes are often tender and may persist for weeks or months following an acute inflammatory process. Lymphomas or other malignancies rarely occur in this area. Enlarged periauricular lymph nodes usually herald otitis externa. They can easily be differentiated from enlargement of the parotid gland, which covers the angle of the mandible.

Sebaceous cysts Older children may develop sebaceous cysts in the face and neck region that may become infected. There is NO CLEAR EVIDENCE to support the argument that sebaceous cysts in children should be removed because they have a tendency to become larger and more troublesome in later life.

Neck

Lymphadenopathy Submandibular lymph nodes are found to be enlarged and palpable in virtually every child in the 2- to 10-year-old age group. Most commonly, the two lymph nodes found about 3 centimeters below the mastoid process in infants and children are brought to the physician's attention. Enlargement of these lymph nodes is almost always due to either a viral or a bacterial infection in the throat. Lymphadenopathy secondary to tuberculosis or a fungal infection is extremely rare but should be considered in populations at risk. With the appropriate use of antibiotics, these lymph nodes rarely become abscessed. The approach to treating submandibular lymphadenopathy should be to first treat the infection causing the lymphadenopathy. An acute infection of the lymph nodes may produce marked enlargement, tenderness, and fever. Oral cloxacillin, 100 mg/kg/24 hours, may result in improvement, but, on occasion, the node may become fluctuant, in which case it should be incised and drained by a surgeon. Malignancy in the lymph nodes of the neck is rare and is most likely to occur in children between the ages of 3 and 6. In children younger than 3, the lymph nodes are rarely malignant. Infectious mononucleosis should also be considered as a cause of lymphadenopathy, especially in children more than 1 or 2 years old.

Enlargement of the thyroid Enlargement of the thyroid in children is due either to thyrotoxicosis or to Hashimoto's thyroiditis. Any nodular enlargement of the thyroid should be considered to be malignant until proven otherwise. Thyroid carcinoma is rare in children but has been reported; if a nodule is palpated on the thyroid, the child should be referred to a consultant.

Thorax

Female breast enlargement Hypertrophy of the breasts is not uncommon, even in the first few years of life. Usually there is absence of other signs of sexual development. If other secondary signs of sexual development occur, the child should be referred to an endocrinologist. The enlarged breasts may be slightly tender and the enlargement symmetrical or asymmetrical. Breast enlargement is caused by a hypersensitivity to estrogen or to increased frequency of estrogen pulses. Gynecomastia in males of pubertal age is a source of anxiety but is of no medical significance (see Chapter 25). Isolated precocious breast development in girls who are growing normally, who have no pubic or axillary hair, and who are in all other respects normal need only be watched. The size of the breasts usually remains stable for months to years and may regress spontaneously until normal puberty occurs.

Genitals—Male

In uncircumcised males, adhesions between the foreskin and the glans disappear by the age of 4 or 5. Inflammation of the foreskin is almost always due to the parents' tampering with the foreskin; their attempts to clean underneath the foreskin or to push it back should be discouraged.

Hydrocele If one side of the scrotum is enlarged, readily compressed, and transilluminates, a hydrocele is probably present. Often there may not be a testis palpable within the hydrocele. Surgical repair is indicated if the hyrocele persists beyond 4 to 5 months of age.

Epididymitis and torsion of the testis Epididymitis is often accompanied by fever, malaise, and other signs of inflammation that help make the diagnosis clear. Epididymitis that is diagnosed by a finding of exquisite tenderness and swelling in the epididymis above the testis should provoke suspicion of other congenital abnormalities (4).

Torsion of the testis is a problem that occurs most commonly in post pubertal boys who are very active physically. Complaint of lower abdominal pain is reason for a scrotal examination to rule out the possibility of torsion of the testis. Swelling in the scrotal area occurs early, and later may be accompanied by fever, tenderness, and severe pain. Torsion of the appendix testis may be difficult to differentiate from a testicular torsion. Surgical exploration, preferably within 6 to 12 hours of the onset of pain, is indicated.

Extremities

Paronychia Paronychia is common in childhood. This inflammation originates at the side of one nail after a piece of cuticle has been pulled or a fingernail has been bitten too far. Paronychia usually does not require surgical repair. A simple treatment is to apply a dressing impregnated with petroleum jelly to the fingertip. The dressing should be left in place for 24 to 48 hours,

during which time the paronychia may break and drain. There is SUGGES-
TIVE EVIDENCE that this method obviates the need for surgical drainage (5).
Antibiotic therapy is not usually indicated.

REFERENCES

1. Anderson, G., Smey, P. Current concepts in the management of common urologic problems in children. *Pediatr. Clin. North Am.* 32:1133–1149, 1985.
2. Martin, D. Germinal cell tumors of the testis after orchiopexy. *J. Urol.* 121:422–424, 1979.
3. Reiger, H. Torsion of an intra-abdominal testis. *Surg. Clin. North Am.* 52:371–378, 1972.
4. Karpe, B., Eneroth, P., Ritzon, N. LHRH treatment in unilateral cryptorchism. *J. Pediatr.* 103:892–897, 1983.
5. Koop, C.E. *Visible and Palpable Lesions in Children.* New York: Grune and Stratton, 1976, p. 93–94.

13

EYE PROBLEMS

PREVALENCE

Fewer than 1% of children have congenital strabismus, whereas up to 5% of children have some form of amblyopia due to undiagnosed strabismus (1). Up to 90% of neonates develop mild conjunctivitis secondary to the administration of silver nitrate solution (2). Bacterial and viral conjunctivitis are the most common eye problems in children, but exact incidence figures are not available. Nasolacrimal duct obstruction occurs in about 6% of infants from birth to 4 months (3). Accurate incidence figures for injuries and burns to the eyes are not available: common household agents that cause eye burns in children are listed in Table 13-1.

RED EYE

Narrowing down and diagnosis (Table 13-2)

In the perinatal period, inflammation of the eye is the most significant eye problem. In most jurisdictions in North America, silver nitrate is routinely infused into the eyes of the newborn to prevent gonococcal conjunctivitis, causing mild conjunctivitis. There is NO CLEAR EVIDENCE that this reaction produces significant problems; however, chloramphenicol or erythromycin can be substituted. Silver nitrate–induced conjunctivitis is usually manifested by a minimal, colored (yellow or green) excretion that crusts around the eyelids. Other causes of conjunctivitis in neonates are much rarer but may include gonococcal, chlamydial, or herpetic conjunctivitis due to infections from the birth canal. There is SUGGESTIVE EVIDENCE that the use of erythromycin may be preferable to silver nitrate, since it is effective against chlamydial conjunctivitis (4).

In older children, staphylococcal blepharoconjunctivitis causes irritation, crusty scales on the lid and inflammation of the conjunctiva. This condition is

Table 13-1. Common household agents that cause conjunctival burns

---
Household ammonia
Window cleaner, jewelry cleaner
Scouring cleaners and powders
Deodorizers
Disinfectants
Toilet bowl cleaners
Drain cleaners
Automotive cleaners, degreasing compounds
Whitewall tire cleaners
Automatic diswasher soap
Lime and plaster
Chlorine (swimming pools)
Swimming pool tile cleaner
Bleach

---

often associated with scalp seborrhea. There may occasionally be superficial punctate erosions on the lower third of the cornea. The child will complain of burning irritation in the eye, excessive tearing, and itching.

A hordeolum (sty) is almost always due to a staphylococcal infection of the glands at the base of the hair follicles of the eyelashes. Usually the patient has pain, redness, and localized, purulent small abscess.

A chalazion is a localized swelling of the eyelid caused by obstruction of the meibomian glands, which causes build-up of lipid material in the subcutaneous tissue.

Viral conjunctival infections, known as epidemic conjunctivitis or "pink eye," are usually caused by adenoviruses. These infections are characterized by a watery discharge, inflammation around the eyes, and conjunctivitis. The conjunctivitis can be severe and may include conjunctival hemorrhages.

Management (Table 13-3)

Eye inflammation in the perinatal period, usually caused by silver nitrate drops, requires no treatment other than soaking with warm water or gentle wiping of the eyes to clear away the crusts. Rarely, there may be development of a mucopurulent discharge, which should be investigated using appropriate cultures and then treated with appropriate topical solutions.

If staphylococcal blepharitis is diagnosed, topical sulfonamides are the drugs of choice, accompanied by hot compresses three to five times daily. The preferred medication is sodium sulfanilamide drops or ophthalmic cream, applied every 4 to 6 hours for 3 to 5 days. The condition is highly infectious, and parents and family should be warned about this. Topical steroids should not be used to reduce inflammation because of the risk of potentiating herpes simplex as well as other viral and fungal infections if they are causing the blepharitis.

Table 13-2. Red eye: Narrowing down the problem

	Etiology		
Symptom	Bacterial	Viral	Foreign body
Discharge from eye	Mucopurulent	Clear	Clear
Irritation or pain	General irritation	General irritation	Pain (focal)
Inflammation of eyelids	Often inflamed, with blepharitis	Minimal erythema	None
Change in visual acuity	Some blurring	Minimal effect	Varies according to site of foreign body

Chlamydial infections respond best to tetracycline, which can be used topically, but its use is contraindicated in neonates. Topical chloramphenicol drops or cream may also be used for chlamydia conjunctivitis. Gonococcal conjunctivitis should be treated with systemic penicillin and topical chloramphenicol cream.

The best treatment for a hordeolum is warm compresses to soften the abscess. Local antibiotics are relatively ineffective. Systemic antibiotics are not indicated unless there is evidence of cellulitis.

The most effective management of a chalazion is application of frequent hot compresses to soften the overlying tissues. Surgical excision may be necessary after 2 to 3 weeks if conservative treatment fails.

Treatment of viral conjunctivitis is supportive. Hot soaks may be soothing, but as yet no antibiotics or antiviral agents have been found to be effec-

Table 13-3. Red eye: Treatment

	Etiology			
Treatment	Bacterial	Viral	Foreign body	Silver nitrate
Hot soaks	Indicated	Indicated	Not helpful	Indicated
Antibiotic solutions	Indicated	Not helpful	Not helpful	Not helpful
Eye patch	Contraindicated	Contraindicated	Helpful for 24 hours if conjunctival or corneal injury	Not indicated
Topical analgesics	Not indicated	Not indicated	For pain from conjunctival or corneal tears	Not indicated

tive. The most important consideration is the prevention of the spread of this highly infectious condition. Such precautions as keeping separate the contaminated washcloths and the careful disposal of all items that have come in contact with the infected area are as important as the personal hygiene of the affected child. Frequent hand-washing of the caretaker is very important.

STRABISMUS

All infants between 1 and 6 months of age should be carefully screened (see Chapter 14, Preventive Health Examinations) for strabismus. Strabismus is defined as a misalignment of the eyes in any direction. In 1- to 6-month-olds, congenital or infantile esotropia is the most common cause of readily visible strabismus. The most accurate office procedures for identifying strabismus include (a) a patch cover test conducted by covering up one eye and watching to see whether the other eye moves "over" to fix on a specific point, (b) an alternating patch test—a patch cover test on one eye and then the other, or (c) the simplest test, fixation of a single light beam on the pupil area to determine if the light reflex is visible at the same place in each pupil. Intermittent esotropia or accommodative esotropia is also common in infants less than 6 months old. The binocular action of the eyes is usually fused, but on occasion there is so-called "wandering eye." One of the most useful ways to detect this phenomenon is to ask the parents if they have ever observed a wandering or lazy eye.

There is FIRM EVIDENCE that an early referral of the child with congenital esotropia to an ophthalmologist for possible surgical intervention can alter the outcome of the disease in terms of fusion of the eyes and visual acuity. Infants with this condition should be identified well before they are 6 months old and referred for assessment. Amblyopia and strabismus of the nonfixed kind should be looked for until 6 years of age, as the late onset of strabismus can be managed with an eye patch or glasses, and, again, early detection is important to prevent blindness in one of the eyes.

TEARING

Contrary to popular belief, tears are produced in the eyes at birth; however, since the amount of liquid produced is small during the first months of life, tears do not normally well up in the eyes. After 3 months of age, it is not uncommon for partial obstruction of the nasolacrimal duct to become apparent. This will cause continual welling up of tears in the eye and possibly chronic or recurrent infection. Between 4 and 8 months of age, in 80% of children with nasolacrimal duct obstruction, the problem spontaneously resolves. This may be aided by advising the parent to compress the nasal lacrimal duct, milking the duct toward the nose, two or three times a day. If, after 6 to 8 months of age, there is no improvement of flow through the duct, then the child should be referred to an ophthamologist.

VISUAL LOSS OR IMPAIRMENT

Difficulties with visual acuity are often noticed in children when they start school, usually between the ages of 4 and 7 years. Although problems of visual acuity often go undetected prior to school admission, they maybe detected at 3 years of age by testing the child's vision using eye charts with symbols or cartoon characters. Simply asking the parents how close the child sits to the television or how close to the eyes the child holds a book or magazine is a crude but useful method of determining visual acuity. A teacher will often become aware that a child is having visual or learning difficulties. Every child who has any type of behavior difficulty at school should undergo a visual assessment as part of the prelimary investigation. Problems of myopia are most common in the primary-school-aged group, and children may require glasses or contact lenses.

Sudden loss of vision in a child for unexplained reasons is exceptionally rare and should be immediately investigated by a consultant. Problems such as retinal artery thrombosis are exceptionally rare in children under the age of 15. Screening for visual acuity problems in children aged 4 to 5 is especially important to prevent their frustration in school studies, and there is SUGGESTIVE EVIDENCE of the benefits of this procedure (5).

EYE INJURIES

A careful history of the onset of the injury will likely determine whether the injury was direct or indirect. Severe, direct injuries secondary to a blow to the eyeball include a blowout fracture, a hemorrhagic hyphema or hemorrhage into the eye, or an injury to the conjunctiva. Visual acuity must be assessed immediately and then monitored frequently to detect deterioration. Careful examination of extraocular movements and funduscopic examination of the eye will determine if there are problems affecting the extraocular muscles, a possible blowout fracture, or introcular hemorrhages. There is FIRM EVIDENCE that children participating in hockey, racket sports, or baseball should wear appropriate eye protection to prevent eye injuries (6).

FOREIGN BODIES

Foreign bodies can be particularly difficult to detect and isolate in a child's eye. The history is of particular importance. If a foreign body is suspected, a very careful examination to reveal any laceration entry points in the cornea or conjunctiva must be made. A history of irritation of the cornea or conjunctiva should also raise suspicion that there is a foreign body in the eye. Use of fluorescein dye and careful slit-lamp examination of the conjunctiva may be necessary. If these examinations do not reveal the foreign body, radiographs and recently developed ultrasound procedures may be helpful in locating a foreign body inside the eye. These procedures may or may not be feasible in the family physician's office or hospital emergency department; they may require an ophthamologist's assistance.

CHEMICAL BURNS, IRRITATION

A wide variety of chemicals can irritate the cornea and conjunctiva, and the irritation may progress to corneal or conjunctival slough burns or damage. Immediate first aid, consisting of profuse washing of the eyes with water, is the most important step in any kind of chemical burn to the eyes. Alkali burns are most dangerous because they penetrate the cornea and anterior chamber more rapidly than do acid burns, and they continue to leach the soft tissues of the eye by binding to the lipids of the cellular membranes. Neutralizing solutions are not usually helpful. Copious irrigation initially is the most important step.

Thermal burns seldom involve the cornea and the globe because of reflex eyelid closure and upward rotation of the eye. Severe burns may be caused by flying tobacco ash or metal, which stay in the eye and result in burning and subsequent scarring. As a first-aid procedure in an acute eye burn, a piece of saran wrap with a thin layer of petroleum jelly or mineral oil should be applied to the skin around the orbit, covering the eye with oil and a protective film, until further treatment can be obtained.

Ultraviolet light exposure usually begins to cause pain and irritation about 6 to 10 hours after the exposure. It is most commonly due to sunlamp exposure, excessive sunburn, or, less commonly, exposure to a welding arc. A foreign body sensation is noticed by the patient, along with marked irritation. Treatment is cycloplegic drops (2% homatropine) and semipressure eye patches for 24 hours.

Indirect injuries to the eye are usually secondary to head injuries that cause cerebral edema and papilledema. Direct visualization of the fundus is usually diagnostic. A severe electric shock may cause blindness for 24 to 48 hours. The exact cause is unknown, but the blindness will almost always resolve and 100% vision will be restored after a few days. It is thought that a complete electrical depolarization of the retinal cells is the cause of this problem.

Pain in the eye of a child is usually due to one of the causes already outlined, although periorbital cellulitis should always be considered. This is most likely due to an infection from a superficial laceration near the eye or ethmoid sinusitis, which can progress very rapidly to obliteration of the orbit. Early detection and immediate antibiotic treatment are essential. Any child who complains of pain in the eye with tenderness or redness in the lid or periorbital region, or pain on compression of the eyeball, should be strongly suspected of having this condition and treated as if that were the case, until it is proven otherwise. Cultures of local exudates and blood cultures should be taken. The child should be hospitalized and given intravenous antibiotics effective against *Haemophilus influenzae* until cultures and bacterial sensitivities are known. Because periorbital cellulitis may lead to cavernous sinus thrombosis and death, pediatric and ophthalmologic consultations are recommended.

REFERENCES

1. Reinecke, R. Current concepts in ophthalmology: Strabismus. *N. Engl. J. Med.* 300: 1139–1141, 1979.
2. Friendly, D. Ophthalmia neonatorum. *Pediatr. Clin. North Am.* 30:1033–1042, 1983.
3. Harley, R. Disease of the lacrimal apparatus. *Pediatr. Clin. North Am.* 30:1159–1166, 1983.
4. Bernstein, G.A., Davis, J.P., Katcher, M.L. Prophylaxis of neonatal conjunctivitis: An analytic review. *Clin. Pediatr.* 21:545–550, 1982.
5. Hall, S., Pugh, A., Hall, D. Vision screening in the under 5's. *Br. Med. J.* 285:1096–1098, 1982.
6. Vinger, P. The incidence of eye injuries in sports. *Int. Ophthalmol. Clin.* 21:21–25, 1981.

14

PREVENTIVE HEALTH EXAMINATIONS

A screening procedure can be defined as a procedure or test that detects an illness early in an asymptomatic person. The procedure is desirable only if there exists an intervention that will alter the natural history of the disease. Preventive health examinations (well-baby examinations) are the most frequently performed examinations in primary care practice. The purpose of the preventive health examination is threefold: (a) to reassure and educate the parents, (b) to conduct appropriate screening tests or procedures, and (c) to conduct appropriate immunization. Screening and case-finding procedures should be conducted prenatally and perinatally and at various other periods in childhood and adolescence. A positive screening test must be reconfirmed before any conclusive diagnosis should be made.

The selection of appropriate preventive health or screening procedures in a primary care practice is complex. Proper evaluation of effective screening procedures requires the consideration of many factors. Some of the basic criteria for effective screening procedures include

1. Is the test or procedure acceptable to both the patient and the physician?
2. Is there an effective ntervention that will alter the natural history of the disease for the patient's benefit?
3. How specific and sensitive are the tests? Detailed methods of calculating specificity and sensitivity of all types of tests are readily available (2).
4. Is the test cost-effective? Some tests such as phenylketonuria screening may have to be done thousands of times to detect one case. However, the prevention of mental retardation in a child compensates for that in both human and monetary terms.
5. What is the burden of mortality, morbidity, and suffering prevented by early detection of an illness? This assessment must consider quality of life for the individual.

In this chapter these five criteria have been used to critically assess the selection of preventive health and screening procedures for three different age groups: prenatal, to prevent problems in the fetus and newborn; newborn up to 1 year of age; and childhood through adolescence. Management of labor and delivery are not included in this discussion. Although many people might find the recommendations given in this chapter incomplete, we are attempting to assess the value of specific procedures and the quality of evidence supporting the use of these procedures.

PRENATAL (TABLE 14–1)

Prenatal care has become increasingly important as our understanding of the causes of fetal abnormalities has improved. In high-risk pregnancies, detection of fetal abnormalities by amniocentesis or ultrasound between 4 and 18 weeks allows parents to choose therapeutic abortion.

The most significant disorder detectable by amniocentesis is Down's syndrome. The incidence of this condition rises as the maternal age increases over 25 (Figure 14-1). If a mother has already given birth to a child with Down's syndrome, the recurrence rate is 1 to 1.5%, depending on maternal age (1A). Other abnormalities include trisomy 18 and trisomy 13 syndromes and miscellaneous autosomal anomalies. Assessment of the family history of both parents is an important part of the first examination in pregnancy and, in fact, should be part of counseling at the time of marriage. A genogram should be developed at this time and added to the family's clinical record.

Rubella syndrome

Rubella syndrome involves a variety of congenital anomalies. Up to 50% of women who have rubella infection in the first month of pregnancy, 22% in the

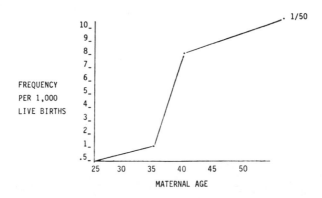

Figure 14-1. Frequency of Down's syndrome per 1,000 live births according to maternal age.

Table 14-1. Prenatal care: Conception to labor

Problem	Narrowing down procedure	Confirmation of diagnosis	Management
Down's syndrome, other known genetic abnormalities	Genetic counseling of high-risk mothers— > 35 years, family history of genetic problems	Amniocentesis at 14 weeks if therapeutic abortion is an option	Therapeutic abortion if acceptable to parents
Rubella syndrome	Prior to conception, assess rubella antibody titer; immunize and confirm effect	Rubella antibody titer early in pregnancy	If significant rise in antibody titer in first trimester, consider therapeutic abortion
Fetal alcohol syndrome	Reduce alcohol intake to 1 oz. or less per day prior to and during pregnancy	Abnormalities usually only detected after birth, e.g., mental retardation, congenital heart disease, abnormal facies	Control or elimination of alcohol ingestion; > 6 oz. of alcohol a day produces syndrome in 50% of babies
Teratogenic drugs	Advise pregnant woman not to use over-the-counter or prescription drugs without assessment of risk by physician	Assessment using appropriate references regarding teratogenic drugs	Therapeutic abortion if high risk before 12 weeks of pregnancy
Malnutrition of mother that adversely affects fetus	Advise about adequate diet; monitor maternal weight gain and fetal growth curve	Evidence of fetal growth retardation	Improved maternal diet
Gestational diabetes mellitus	2-hour PC blood glucose at 20–24 weeks; urine glucose on prenatal visits	Modified glucose tolerance test at 24 weeks of gestation	Management of high-risk pregnancy with careful monitoring and early delivery
Risk assessment of pregnancy	Detection of high risk	Consultation with high-risk pregnancy expert	Varies depending on problem
Maternal smoking	Ask mother about smoking habit	Estimate of fetal growth	Smoking cessation or management of low-birth-weight baby

second month, 10% in the third month, and 6 to 10% in the third to sixth month give birth to infants suffering from the rubella syndrome. The syndrome resulting from infection in the first trimester is characterized by congenital cataracts, congenital heart anomalies, mental retardation, microcephaly, and deafness. The syndrome resulting from infection in the second trimester usually is marked by mental and motor retardation and deafness. Ideally, all women, before they become sexually active, should have their rubella antibody titer determined (1).

Rubella immunization is most effective before a child reaches age 12. After 12 years of age, there is decreasing likelihood that the antibody titer will rise after immunization. In a 25-year-old woman who has no antibodies and who is given the RV27 attenuated rubella virus immunization, there is a 25% chance that the antibody titer will not rise subsequent to the immunization. However, the lack of antibody titer rise may or may not indicate lack of immunity. It is important, in females over age 12, to measure antibody titers 6 weeks post-immunization to demonstrate that the immunization has been effective (2,3). The antibody titer should be assessed early in pregnancy so that if, by chance, the woman is exposed to rubella early in her pregnancy, an antibody titer rise will be measurable. If there is a threefold rise in the antibody titer during pregnancy, especially with a history of exposure or rash, then the woman should be informed of the risks and offered the option of a therapeutic abortion. (4–6).

Fetal alcohol syndrome

The fetal alcohol syndrome has only recently been described. Further research is necessary to understand what alcohol dosage causes development of the syndrome. It is not known if the time of consumption of alcohol during pregnancy is important. It has been documented that women who consume more than 6 ounces of alcohol a day during their pregnancy have as much as a 50 to 60% chance of delivering a child suffering from fetal alcohol syndrome (7). The syndrome is characterized by specific facial characteristics, congenital heart anomalies, and mental retardation. The percentage of offspring with the syndrome of women who consume less than 6 ounces of alcohol a day is not known.

Currently, the most conservative policy is to recommend that the mother consume no alcohol from the time of conception onward, since the dose relationship between alcohol and anomalous development is unknown. However, there is NO CLEAR EVIDENCE that less than 3 ounces of alcohol a day results in defects (8). There is no method of detecting the abnormalities associated with the fetal alcohol syndrome prenatally, as they rarely involve gross congenital anomalies that would be detectable by ultrasound. Mothers should be informed of the risks involved in consuming large quantities of alcohol and the possible risks of consuming small amounts of alcohol during pregnancy (7). Patient education is the only method of dealing with this problem. There is SUGGESTIVE EVIDENCE of a fivefold decrease in alcohol consumption in early pregnancy when women are aware of the syndrome (9).

Teratogenic drugs

Different drugs are variably teratogenic. The most commonly known teratogenic drugs include thalidomide, aminopterin, methotrexate, trimethoprim-sulfamethoxasole, clotrimazole, androgens, and Acutane. The handbook for prescribing during pregnancy (10) should always be available to the physician to aid in assessing the risk of any drug to a pregnant woman. Each individual case must be evaluated for the risk of the adverse effect on the fetus of high fever or extreme illness in the mother relative to the known or potential teratogenic risk of the drug. Drug interactions during pregnancy are not well understood; therefore, minimizing drug use is the most prudent policy. During the office visit when pregnancy is being planned or during the first prenatal visit, the woman should be informed that no drugs, either over-the-counter or by prescription, should be taken without consulting the physician. If, as often occurs, potentially teratogenic drugs were given to a woman before she knew she was pregnant, then a decision will have to be made as to whether the risk of teratogenicity is unacceptable and whether the woman wants a therapeutic abortion because of that risk. Each case will have to be judged on its own merits.

When providing continuous care to a woman who is planning a pregnancy, a discussion about drug use should take place prior to the pregnancy so that during the period when the woman is at risk of becoming pregnant, she will not take drugs that could interfere with the pregnancy.

Malnutrition

Significant malnutrition in a pregnant woman may adversely affect the fetus. There is FIRM EVIDENCE that hypoproteinemic diets during pregnancy can reduce development of nerve tissue in the fetus and may have long-term adverse results. Dietary counseling and instruction, combined with monitoring of both maternal and fetal growth curves, are important during pregnancy. It is especially important to monitor the fetal growth curve (Figure 14-2). Early evidence of fetal growth retardation should prompt careful assessment of the mother's diet and an increase in the protein content of the diet as well as appropriate vitamin supplementation. There is NO CLEAR EVIDENCE that vitamin deficiencies in North American diets cause significant fetal problems. Although many physicians advise the use of iron supplements throughout pregnancy to prevent anemia in the mother, there is NO CLEAR EVIDENCE of a need to overcome the net loss of about 1,500 milligrams of iron throughout pregnancy and delivery in a well-nourished woman. There is as yet NO

CLEAR EVIDENCE that folic acid or other vitamin supplementation in the average North American woman is likely to alter the outcome of pregnancy.

Gestational diabetes mellitus

The perinatal mortality rate in undetected gestational diabetes is between 5 and 8%. If an appropriate screening program is implemented, 25 in 1,000 women screened will be found to have gestational diabetes. There is FIRM EVIDENCE that early delivery and increased surveillance during pregnancy will reduce the risk for the fetus. The two most significant screening procedures during pregnancy are obtaining the family history and monitoring the mother's urine. Any family history of diabetes places the pregnant woman in a high-risk group. Throughout pregnancy, assessment of the urine for glucose on each visit is worthwhile. Any woman with two 2+ urine tests for glucose and a significant family history should undergo a glucose tolerance test immediately. Recently, some obstetricians have advocated that all pregnant women undergo a modified glucose tolerance test at 24 weeks of pregnancy (11). NO CLEAR EVIDENCE of the efficacy of this procedure exists in the current literature.

Management of the gestational diabetic who is detected at any stage of pregnancy includes careful monitoring of blood glucose levels on a weekly or biweekly basis. The pregnancy should be managed in collaboration with a high-risk pregnancy unit or consultant.

Maternal smoking

Any pregnant woman who smokes more than two or three cigarettes per day should be told of the risk of adverse effects for the fetus. These include higher perinatal mortality, significantly lower average birth weight, and, now, suggestions of perceptual and other developmental problems in the young child (12). The pregnant woman should be strongly encouraged to stop smoking. Unfortunately, there is NO CLEAR EVIDENCE that pressure to reduce or stop smoking is particularly effective during pregnancy, although there are numerous anecdotal reports of success.

Risk assessment of pregnancy

The purpose of assessing risk early in pregnancy is to detect women who are at high risk of having perinatal difficulties or difficulties that place the fetus at high risk during pregnancy. This is especially important for physicians who are practicing in rural or remote areas when the implications are that the woman would have to be admitted to a high-risk center during the third trimester. There is FIRM EVIDENCE that detection and early referral to a high-risk management center is beneficial to the fetus. Using a simple risk assessment table, the level of risk can be readily estimated and appropriate actions taken early in the pregnancy to prevent serious complications later (Figure 14-2).

NEWBORN TO 1 YEAR (TABLE 14-2)

How often a newborn should be examined through to 1 year of age is a topic of considerable controversy. As long as the child is healthy at the time of delivery, most hospitals recommend that the child be assessed within 24 hours of delivery in some detail as well as prior to discharge from hospital. The frequency with which the child is then assessed and by whom has long been controversial. Gilbert et al. (13) conducted a randomized trial assessing five and ten well-baby visits in the first 2 years of life. Several outcome measures were used to determine if, after 2 years, any differences could be noted in the two groups in both frequency of illness and abnormalities that had gone undetected. A pediatrician who was blind to which group each baby was in assessed all 400 participants after 2 years. No significant differences were noted in either group. In spite of this FIRM EVIDENCE, many family physicians and pediatricians recommend that a child be assessed as frequently as once a month for the first year of life (13). Most physicians now assess children at 1 month of age after their initial perinatal assessments, and at 2, 4, 6, 9, and 12 months. The strongest argument for this program is that it corresponds with the immunization program that most physicians follow. On this basis, the 9-

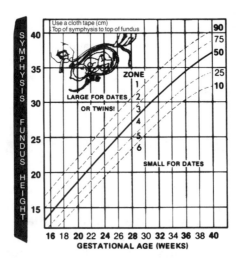

Figure 14-2. Monitoring fetal growth. Zones 1 and 6 are high risk. A change of two zones up or down may be significant. (Courtesy of the Ontario Medical Association.)

Table 14-2. Newborn and well-baby care to 1 year of age

Problem	Narrowing down procedure	Confirmation of diagnosis	Management
Gross congenital anomalies: imperforate anus, absent limbs, spina bifida, cleft palate, esophageal atresia, club foot	General physical examination, including orifices, mouth	Appropriate probing or radiograph	Appropriate surgical intervention
Congenital hip dislocation	Hip click test; all well-baby exams prior to walking	Triple diapering followed by frog leg radiograph	Appropriate splint
Strabismus	Patch test or light reflex test; all well-child exams	Ophthalmologic assessment	Surgical correction
Congenital heart defect	Auscultation for murmurs; assessment for cyanosis or respiratory problems; all well-baby exams	Appropriate non-invasive tests or heart catheterization	Surgical correction
Deafness	Clap test; parental assessment of hearing; all well-baby exams	Audiology assessment; auditory evoked potentials	Hearing aid and speech therapy from earliest age of detection
Child abuse	Assessment of parental social support, attitudes, and risk	Assessment of injuries; physical exam, radiography; social agency	Appropriate intervention to protect child
Abnormal growth	Growth curve chart to monitor child development and physical well-being	Precise assessment; investigation appropriate to situation	Investigation appropriate to diagnosis
Phenylketonuria	PKU screening by heel-prick blood test	Measurement of serum phenylalanine	Phenylalanine-restricted diet
Congenital hypothyroidism (cretinism)	T_4 or TSH levels, by heel-prick blood test, usually 2–3 days post partum	Serum T_4 and TSH levels	Thyroxine supplementation

T_4, thyroxine; TSH, thyroid-stimulating hormone.

month visit could be discontinued; however, some physicians argue that 9 months is an important time to assess nutrition and the prewalking status of the child.

Based on the data of Gilbert et al. (13) and the most commonly used immunization program, the schedule outlined in Table 14-3 is recommended, assuming the baby is in good health and is not at high risk (1).

The following procedures should be carried out in the newborn or on well-baby visits up to 1 year of age. Each has been assessed critically and is supported by FIRM EVIDENCE in the current literature to justify its use in routine screening.

Gross congenital anomalies

The newborn baby should be assessed in the delivery room or within a few hours of birth with the purpose of detecting gross congenital anomalies for which early intervention is indicated. Congenital anomalies that are significant include spina bifida, genital anomalies, cleft palate, talipes equinovarus, and esophageal atresia (Table 14-4). Early detection of these anomalies will prevent serious deterioration of the infant's condition prior to appropriate surgical intervention. A physical assessment of the body, spine, and limbs (for club feet), visualization of the eyes, and examination of the roof of the mouth are important. Early detection of rectovaginal fistulas or an imperforate anus is also important to minimize adverse effects in the neonate.

Congenital hip dislocation

Congenital hip dislocations occur in approximately 1.1 to 1.7 times in every 1,000 live births (14–16). The hip dislocation is more common in males than females and is best detected by flexing the hips to 90°, then maximally abducting them and performing the Ortolani maneuver. This procedure is most likely to be positive at about 3 to 6 weeks post partum. Maternal progesterone

Table 14-3. Immunization and visit schedule

2 months	Diphtheria, pertussis, tetanus (DPT) with or without Salk vaccine; if without, oral polio vaccine (OPV)
4 months	DPT with or without Salk vaccine; if without, OPV
6 months	DPT with or without Salk vaccine; if without, OPV
12–15 months	Measles, mumps, rubella
18 months	DPT booster (with polio if Salk used)
5 years	DPT booster (with polio if Salk used)
12 years	Rubella titer assessment or rubella vaccine
14–16 years	dT with polio if Salk used

Table 14-4. Incidence of common congenital anomalies

	Frequency per live births	Recurrence risk after 1 affected child
Spina bifida (anencephaly)	1–2.5/1,000	1/25
Pyloric stenosis (previously seen in male relative)	1/200	1/15
Cleft lip, palate	1/1,000	1/25
Talipes equinovarus	1/1,000	1/50
Ventricular septal defect	1/1,000	1/25
Pyloric stenosis in female (with a history in a female relative)	1/1,000	1/25

has the effect of softening the ligaments that surround the hip joint and reducing the likelihood of a positive "hip click" immediately post partum. Op-
timally, the test should be done on every visit before the child walks. This approach will increase the sensitivity of the test. If congenital hip dislocation is
suspected, the baby should be triple-diapered and reassessed in 4 weeks. If
the suspicion remains, then referral of the infant to an orthopedist is important. There is FIRM EVIDENCE that early intervention with a Salter splint
prevents the development of problems that require extensive surgery and
have less than ideal outcomes (1).

Strabismus

Manifest or latent strabismus is present in 6 to 7% of infants at birth. If a significant congenital problem is detected prior to 6 months of age, then an
ophthalmologic consultation is necessary. One hundred percent fusion of
the vision in two eyes will occur with therapy for congenital strabismus prior
to 6 months of age. Between 5 and 9 years of age, the likelihood of obtaining
full fusion decreases to the point where vision in one eye will be blocked out
permanently. Use of either a patch cover test or direct visual observation of
the light reflex in the pupils is the appropriate procedure. This assessment
should be carried out during every visit prior to 6 months of age. The
mother's help in observing that the child's eyes are always straight or that
they "wander" should be solicited at the first well-baby visit (1). See Chapter
13, Eye Problems.

Congenital heart defects

The most common and significant congenital heart defect detected by auscultation is ventricular septal defect. The incidence of VSD is 1.5 to 2 per 1,000

live births. Twenty to fifty percent of VSDs are detected by repeated ausculta-tion of the heart for murmurs. The cyanotic child will be diagnosed at birth or shortly thereafter, if careful observation and inspections are made post par-tum. Murmurs have to be differentiated from the functional flow murmurs that are very common in infants (see Chapter 9). A suspected VSD should be investigated with a chest radiograph, electrocardiogram, and referral for a cardiologic opinion. Early intervention may prevent pulmonary hyperten-sion and extend life expectancy (1).

Hearing impairment

Congenital hearing loss may be secondary to rubella syndrome or a variety of other drug-induced or congenital problems. One in 1,000 babies is pro-foundly deaf, whereas as many as 3% of school-aged children have impair-ment of hearing significant enough to require special school programs. Early detection of profound deafness and introduction of special programs and hearing aids can improve the child's communication skills significantly. A negative result of the so-called clap test, in which sharp noises produced out of the visual range of the child do not elicit a startle response, suggests the need for further assessment. The mother's assistance can also be solicited — she can observe the child's response to sounds at home. The clap test should be repeated on every visit up to 1 year. A test for brainstem auditory evoked potentials can be carried out at birth in babies at high risk for deafness or later if the physician or parents are suspicious. Special hearing aids and communi-cation programs should be started as soon as deafness is diagnosed. (See Chapter 3, Ear Problems.)

Child abuse

Table 14-5 lists the predictors of family situations that indicate high risk of child abuse. Early detection of high-risk parents and monitoring the well-being of the child may lead to early intervention in a situation that could otherwise result in serious harm to the child. Even in low-risk situations, fre-quent injuries characteristic of child abuse should increase the physician's suspicions. Notification of appropriate agencies is mandatory in many juris-dictions when there is suspicion of child abuse (17). Since questioning either the parents or the child about possible abuse is a very sensitive matter, there are several possible approaches to screening. Many physicians advocate a "third person" approach to questioning. An example of a question is, "Par-ents in your situation may get very upset by their child's behavior and resort to shaking or slapping the child. How often do you feel that way?" Or, "Most parents get tired and exasperated with crying children. Have you ever be-come angry and struck the child?" (See the section on child battering in Chap-ter 24.)

Table 14-5. Risk factors for child abuse

Unstable background of mother
    Early separation from parents
    Foster homes
    Divorce
    Unhappy childhood, including beating, neglect, and deprivation
    Drugs
    Alcohol
    Lack of social support

Child of the "wrong" sex

Parent feels child does not love him or her

Multiple calls for help, i.e., emergency room visits for illness, etc.

Abnormal expectations for the child

High stress level in the home

Mother under age 24 and unmarried

Failure to thrive

Abnormal growth

Monitoring of a child's height and weight on each visit in the first year of life is a traditional procedure (Table 14-6). Deviations above or below the third or ninety-seventh percentile suggest that there may be a significant problem. Children who have been progressing normally but who experience a major change in percentile levels may have a serious underlying disease. Lack of progress in height is more suggestive of hormonal deficiency than are changes in weight. A child who has been in the appropriate percentile as far as weight for height and whose weight then increases should be evaluated. Discussions of growth and weight problems are contained in Chapter 19. The most common causes of an increase in weight include over-feeding, under-exercising, and genetic factors. The most common causes of failure to progress sufficiently in weight include feeding problems, environment deprivation, and chronic underlying disease.

Phenylketonuria

Although the incidence of phenylketonuria is very low (between 1 in 10,000 and 1 in 15,000 live births), early detection prevents severe mental retardation. The test is relatively simple and inexpensive and therefore is definitely a cost-effective procedure. One of the problems involved in PKU testing is that the optimal time for a significant level of phenylalanine to occur in the blood is after the infant has had a reasonable supply of dietary protein; with the trend toward discharging newborns early from the hospital, there may be false-negative PKU test results. It may therefore be necessary to have the test

Table 14-6. Care of children from 1 year on

Problem	Narrowing down procedure	Confirmation of diagnosis	Management
Abnormal growth and development	Monitor milesones of (table) weight and height	Investigate deviations from milestones or growth curve, <3rd or >97th percentile	Management depending on problem
Child abuse	Child behavior, injuries; assessment of risk (table)	Assessment of home situation, social situation	Appropriate intervention to protect child

done at home or the office a few days after discharge. There is FIRM EVI-DENCE that intervention within 3 to 4 weeks with a phenylalanine-restricted diet will prevent the serious outcomes of phenylketonuria in the child (1).

Congenital hypothyroidism

Congenital hypothyroidism occurs in approximately 1 in 15,000 to 1 in 20,000 live births. The test is a simple thyroxine level obtained by drawing blood in a heel-prick sample from the infant in the nursery. Confirmation of the test result if an abnormality is detected in the initial test is by determining both thyroxine and thyroid-stimulating hormone levels. There is FIRM EVI-DENCE that early detection of this syndrome and replacement thyroxine therapy usually reduce the serious complications of cretinism (1).

Immunization

Immunization continues to be the cornerstone of preventive medicine. Although each vaccine and the sequence in which it is given are the subjects of many studies about effectiveness and side effects, the program outlined in Table 14-1 is currently the most widely accepted immunization schedule. Availability of vaccines and regional use of a variety of combinations of vaccines will require individual adaptation of the program outlined (1). Recently, there has been controversy over the use of pertussis vaccine, as the vaccine has been known to cause severe reactions, including seizures, encephalopathy, and death. Table 14-7 outlines the evidence that the benefits of the vaccine far outweigh the risks. There is FIRM EVIDENCE that there is no relationship between sudden infant death syndrome and the pertussis vaccine (18).

Table 14-7. Risk of complications after pertussis vaccine compared with those of whooping cough

| | Risk of occurence | | Relative risk ratio |
Problem	Vaccine	Disease	(Disease/vaccine)
Seizures	1/1,750	1/25–1/250	7–70/1
Vascular collapse	1/1,750	Not known	Not known
Encephalopathy	1/110,000	1/1,000–1/4,000	28–110/1
Permanent brain damage	1/310,000	1/2,000–1/8,000	39–155/1
Death	1/1,000,000	1/200–1/1,000	1,000–5,000/1

SUMMARY

Screening and preventive health examinations for the fetus during pregnancy and for the infant after birth are extremely important, since early detection of preventable or treatable problems can ensure a lifetime free of unnecessary morbidity or early mortality.

REFERENCES

1. Periodic Health Examination. Report of Task Force to the Conference of Deputy
   Ministers of Health. Department of Supply and Services, Ottawa, 1980, pp. 24–
   30, 31–32, 49–50.
1A. Burgio, G.R., Fraccar, O.M., Tiepoco, L., Wolf, U., *Trisomy 21.* Springer-Verlag,
   New York, 1981, p. 214.
2. Balfour, H., Groth, K., Edelman, C. RA27/3 rubella vaccine. A four-year follow
   up. *Am. J. Dis. Child.* 134:350–353, 1980.
3. Balfour, H., Groth, K., Edelman, C. Rubella viremia and antibody response to
   rubella vaccination and re-immunization. *Lancet* 1:8229:1078–1080, 1981.
4. Gershon, J. Life attenuated rubella virus vaccine: Comparison of responses to
   HPV-77-DE5 and RA27/3 strains. *Am. J. Med. Sci.* 279:95–97, 1980.
5. Brunell, P.A., Weigle, K., Murphy, M.D., Shehab, Z., Cobb, E. Antibody response following measles-mumps-rubella vaccine under conditions of custom-
   ary use. *J.A.M.A.* 250:1409–1412, 1983.
6. Coulombe, L., Rosser, W. Can we prevent an increase in the incidence of congenital rubella syndrome in the next decade? *Can. Med. Assoc. J.* 125:37–40, 1981.
7. Sokol, R. Alcohol and abnormal outcomes of pregnancy. *Can. Med. Assoc. J.*
   125:143–148, 1981.
8. Ashley, M. Symposium: Alcohol and the foetus. *Can. Med. Assoc. J.* 125:141–142,
   1981.
9. Rosett, H., Weiner, L. Identifying and treating pregnant patients at risk from alcohol. *Can. Med. Assoc. J.* 125:149–153, 1981.
10. Berkowitz, R., Coustan, D., Mochizuke, J. *Handbook for Prescribing Medication dur-
    ing Pregnancy.* Boston: Little, Brown, 1981.
11. O'Sullivan, J., Mahan, C., Charles, D. Screening criteria for high risk gestational
    diabetic patients. *Am. H. Obstet. Gynecol.* 116:895–900, 1973.
12. Gussela, J., Fried, P.A. Effects of maternal social smoking and drinking on off-
    spring at 13 months. *Neurobehav. Toxicol. Terotol.* 6:13–17, 1984.
13. Gilbert, J., Feldman, W., Seigal, L. How many well baby visits are necessary in the
    first two years of life? *Can. Med. Assoc. J.* 130:857–861, 1984.
14. Barlow, T. Early diagnosis and treatment of congenital dislocation of the hip joint
    in the newborn. *J. Bone Joint Surg.* 44-B:292–297, 1962.
15. Rosen, S. Diagnosis and treatment of congenital dislocation of the hip joint in the
    newborn. *J. Bone Joint Surg.* 44-B:284, 1962.
16. Bell, M., Fraser J. The incidence of dislocated hips in Chinese: Prospective study
    of 50,000 newborn examinations. *Orthop. Trans.* 6:467–470, 1982.
17. Shearman, J., Shemilt, R., Magder, D. Potential child abuse. *Canadian Family
    Physician* 22:739–743, 1976.
18. Gold, R. Pertussis and pertussis vaccine. *Canada Diseases Weekly Report* 11:8, 1985.

Growth, Development, and Adaptation

15

COMMON PROBLEMS
IN THE NEWBORN

This chapter reviews the common problems that face the family physician or obstetrician during and immediately after birth of the newborn. The major problems discussed are acute resuscitation, congenital anomalies, respiratory distress, and jaundice.

PREVALENCE

Fewer than 10% of newborns require resuscitative intervention beyond simple suctioning or availability of oxygen. Routine tube suctioning for newborns without breathing problems is not indicated; this procedure produces bradycardia and hypoxia in 10 to 15% of babies (1).

Between 9 and 15% of all deliveries involve meconium staining of the amniotic fluid (2). Approximately 1% of all live births develop respiratory distress syndrome (3). The frequency of this problem rises in direct relation to the prematurity of the baby. The incidence is also higher in babies born by cesarean section, in males, and in newborns who require resuscitation because of perinatal asphyxia. Jaundice occurs in 33 to 50% of healthy newborn babies. Breast-feeding may prolong physiologic jaundice in 1 in 50 to 1 in 200 breast-fed infants. Fewer than 3% of term infants without blood group incompatibility develop bilirubin levels greater than 15 mg/dl. Birth injuries are, fortunately, rare, occurring in approximately 5 in 1000 live births. Fractured clavicle is the most common injury. The prevalences of the most common congenital problems are shown in Table 15-1.

NARROWING DOWN AND MANAGING
RESPIRATORY PROBLEMS

Appropriate measures of resuscitation, when necessary, have a major impact on the infant's future well-being. An effective method of rapidly assessing the

Table 15-1. Incidence of and sex ratio for common malformations

	Incidence per 1,000 live births	Sex ratio (M/F)
Congenital heart malformation	2	1.0
Pyloric stenosis	3	5.0
Spina bifida*	1.0–2.5	2.5
Anencephaly*	2	0.4
Down's syndrome	2	1.0
Cleft palate	1	1.8
Talipes equinovarus	1	2.0
Congenital hip dislocation	1	0.15

Data from ref. 6.

*Spina bifida and anencephaly are often combined statistically as neuronal tube defects. The incidence is lower in North America than in the United Kingdom. In 1980, the incidence of neuronal tube defects was 0.85/1,000 in British Comumbia (7), and, in 1983, 1.65/1,000 live births in the United Kingdom (8).

cardiorespiratory status of the newborn is essential. The most effective tool is the Apgar score (Table 15-2). Traditionally, the score is taken at 1 and 5 minutes after birth, but it may be needed for immediate assessment at the time of delivery of asphyxial babies. In addition, repeated assessments may be required during the first few minutes of life. The 1-minute Apgar score indicates what steps must be taken in resuscitation, while the 5-minute Apgar score predicts the neurological outcome. The Apgar system should be familiar to and used by all personnel involved in obstetrical care. Table 15-3 outlines the expected Apgar scores at specific times after delivery and the steps in resuscitation required if the scores are not met.

Initial suctioning when the baby's head is born should be gentle bulb suction. Studies have provided FIRM EVIDENCE that nasal or pharyngeal tube

Table 15-2. The Apgar score

Characteristic	Apgar score		
	0	1	2
Heart rate	0	< 100	> 100
Respiratory effort	Apnea	Irregular shallow gasping	Vigorous and crying
Color	Pale blue	Pale or blue extremities	Pink
Muscle tone	Absent	Weak, passive tone	Active movement
Reflex irritability	Absent	Grimace	Active avoidance

Data from ref. 9.

suctioning stimulates bradycardia and hypoxia in 10 to 15% of newborns. Gentle bulb suctioning within the first minute of life or prior to the delivery of the shoulders is the procedure advocated (1). If by 1 minute or later the infant is moderately asphyxial, then oxygen should be administered. There is FIRM EVIDENCE that cold, dry oxygen blown directly into the child's nares will stimulate bradycardia and hypoxia, whereas room-warmed, humidified oxygen, blown across the face prevents such adverse effects (2). It is very important to intubate the severely asphyxial infant immediately and to artificially provide a prolonged inspiration as the first breath. This maneuver stimulates the cardiorespiratory system in most cases. There are a number of controversies regarding the use of atropine, sodium bicarbonate, and adrenaline to stimulate breathing. There is NO FIRM EVIDENCE to support or refute the use of any of these drugs in asphyxial newborns.

If there was meconium staining before labor commenced, permanent damage to the lungs and cardiorespiratory system may already have taken place. However, if meconium staining occurs during late labor or delivery,

Table 15-3. Management of acute resuscitation of the newborn on the basis of the Apgar score

Apgar score	Management
Step A—8, 9, 10 (no asphyxia)	1. Gentle suction with bulb syringe only. 2. Maintain body temperature. 3. Conduct brief physical examination. 4. Assign Apgar score.
Step B—5, 6, 7 (mild asphyxia)	1. Repeat gentle suction with bulb syringe. 2. Maintain body temperature. 3. Stimulate breathing by slapping soles of feet or rubbing spine or sternum. 4. Provide enriched oxygen by bag and mask near baby's face. 5. If score rises to 8 +, carry out steps A-3 and A-4. 6. If heart rate falls to below 100, initiate step C.
Step C—3 or 4 (moderate asphyxia)	1. Repeat steps A-1 and 2. Call for help to monitor heart rate, manage airway, provide cardiac massage. 2. Provide a brief trial of stimulation (B-3) and provide pure O_2 by mask for 1 minute only; if no response, proceed to C-3. 3. Ventilate with bag and mask using 100% O_2 and pressure adequate to move chest. Continue until heart rate is > 100, color is pink, and breathing is spontaneous. If chest does not move with ventilation, intubate. 4. If heart rate is < 60, intubate and begin cardiac massage—2 compressions per second.
Step D—1 or 2 (severe asphyxia)	1. Intubate immediately, bag ventilate with 100% O_2 at 40–60 respirations per minute, with pressure moving upper chest. 2. Perform cardiac massage. 3. If heart rate is not > 100 after 2 minutes, insert intravenous umbilical catheter and administer intravenous fluids, starting with $NAHCO_3$–dextrose. 4. Seek pediatric assistance or anesthesia assistance.

meconium aspiration can still be prevented. As soon as there is evidence of meconium staining, tube suctioning of the infant's nose and throat prior to the first gasps and the delivery of the shoulders may clear the meconium from the nares and from the mouth. The adverse effects of meconium aspiration are worse than the risk of inducing hypoxia and bradycardia by tube suctioning. Once the infant is born, there is FIRM EVIDENCE that endotracheal suctioning until all the meconium-stained fluid has been removed from the pharynx and upper trachea will dramatically lower the incidence of aspiration pneumonia, a condition with significant morbidity and mortality (3). Assessment of the amniotic fluid prior to delivery is important to determine whether these steps should be taken at the time of delivery to prevent meconium aspiration.

After acute resuscitation, the most likely cause of respiratory difficulties within minutes up to 2 hours after birth is respiratory distress syndrome. The clinical picture includes intercostal retraction, tachypnea, and expiratory grunts. As the problem worsens, there may be cyanosis, systemic hypotension, and a characteristic chest radiograph.

If the mother is at risk of premature labor or delivery, lecithin/sphingomyelin ratios should be measured, as they have a better than 90% predictive value for infants at risk for respiratory distress syndrome. The management of respiratory distress syndrome has dramatically improved over the last 15 years, with the most significant advance being the appropriate utilization of mechanical ventilators. A newborn on a respirator is best cared for in a neonatal intensive care unit. Physicians anticipating the birth of a baby at risk for respiratory distress syndrome should transfer the mother before delivery to a regional perinatal care center. Should the newborn show the first signs of respiratory distress, he or she should be kept warm, given oxygen, and immediately transferred to a neonatal intensive care unit.

Primary care physicians practicing obstetrics away from a major center should be aware of the FIRM EVIDENCE that betamethasone given to the mother at least 24 hours prior to delivery, before 32 weeks of gestation, significantly reduces mortality from respiratory distress syndrome (4,5). Signs of respiratory difficulty, especially in a premature infant, should be considered respiratory distress syndrome unless there is evidence of another cause, since other conditions, such as pneumothorax, aspiration pneumonia, and pulmonary hypertension, are much less common. Onset of respiratory problems after the first 2 to 3 hours of life makes pneumonia more likely than respiratory distress syndrome.

NARROWING DOWN THE PROBLEM
AND MANAGING CONGENITAL ANOMALIES

Congenital cardiovascular anomalies may be present if tachycardia, tachypnea, and cyanosis persist after the initial resuscitation phase of 5 or 10 minutes. After the first few hours of life, feeding difficulties, excessive perspiration, and dyspnea are also signs of congenital heart disease. Heart murmurs are prominent at birth with some anomalies, while murmurs are heard only after a few days or even weeks of life in other conditions. Table 15-4 shows the prevalences of different congenital heart anomalies. Any newborn child with evidence of congestive heart failure or respiratory distress secondary to cardiac anomalies must be referred to a tertiary care center.

There are several gastrointestinal abnormalities that can occur in the newborn. Any pregnant woman with hydramnios should be considered at risk of giving birth to an infant with an esophageal fistula or atresia. Excessive amniotic fluid is reason to carefully pass a tube into the newborn's stomach in the delivery room to rule out atresia. Any evidence of fistula or atresia requires very careful esophageal and tracheal suctioning to reduce the risk of aspiration pneumonia. The normal newborn should pass meconium within 12 to 24 hours. In cases of obstruction, abdominal distention and vomiting begin within 6 to 12 hours. At the first sign of intestinal obstruction, it is very important that the stomach be decompressed by continuous gastric suctioning to prevent aspiration. An imperforate anus is detected by assessment of the anal area. Meconium ileus secondary to either cystic fibrosis or Hirschsprung's disease is another cause that should be considered in the early investigation of bowel obstruction. If a congenital anomaly of the gastrointestinal tract is suspected, the newborn should be transferred to a tertiary care pediatric facility.

Even with the elimination of hemorrhagic disease of the newborn, rare bleeding events may still be caused by vitamin K deficiency. Hemorrhagic disease of the newborn is caused by an inconsistent amount of ingested vitamin K, combined with the initial sterility of the gut and the 2 to 4 days required for adequate intestinal colonization. Vitamin K precursors are synthesized in the liver. There is adequate vitamin K in the infant's circulation for the first 24 hours of life; thus vitamin K deficiency occurs after the first 24 hours. Virtually all newborn nurseries now administer intramuscular vitamin K either in

Table 15-4. Diagnostic frequency of the most common congenital heart anomalies

	No. per 10,000 live births
Ventricular septal defect	3.45–10
Transposition of the great vessels	2.18
Tetralogy of Fallot	1.96
Coarctation of the aorta	1.65
Hypoplastic left heart	1.63
Patent ductus arteriosus	1.35

Data from ref. 10.

the delivery room or on admission to the newborn nursery. Hemorrhagic problems after 24 hours of age should be considered the result of a failure to administer vitamin K. Most other hemorrhagic conditions of the newborn secondary to hereditary disorders show bleeding within the first 24 hours. Extensive hematological investigation will be necessary to sort out the other rare hemorrhagic diseases.

NARROWING DOWN THE PROBLEM
AND MANAGING JAUNDICE

Hyperbilirubinemia causes considerable anxiety for parents and physicians. Physiological jaundice in the newborn is caused by hemolysis, transient deficiency in liver-conjugating enzymes, and decreased liver uptake of bilirubin, as well as decreased renal excretion. Breast-feeding may also prolong jaundice. Characteristically, with breast-milk jaundice there is a rise in bilirubin after the third day of life. The level may rise to 20 to 25 mg/100 ml by the end of the second week of life. In spite of such high levels of bilirubin, the infant otherwise functions normally. Interruption in nursing will produce a fall in serum bilirubin within 24 to 72 hours. If the bilirubin concentration fails to decline within 3 days, human milk is probably not the cause of the jaundice. After such a fall, resumption of breast-feeding is usually associated with only a slight rise in the bilirubin. Although very high levels of bilirubin may occur in breast-milk jaundice, no cases of kernicterus have been reported. How-

Table 15-5. Guidelines for use of phototherapy in the newborn period

Birth weight (g)	Indications for phototherapy
< 1,500	Start phototherapy during first 24 hours, regardless of bilirubin concentration
1,500–1,999	Without hemolysis, start phototherapy at 10 mg/dl. With hemolysis, start at 8 mg/dl.
2,000–2,499	Without hemolysis, start phototherapy at 12 mg/dl. With hemolysis, start phototherapy at 10 mg/dl
> 2,500	Without hemolysis in healthy infant, withhold until 15 mg/dl. With hemolysis, start phototherapy at 15 mg/dl

	Indications for exchange transfusion (mg/dl bilirubin)					
Birth weight (g)	< 1,000	1,000–1,249	1,250–1,499	1,500–1,999	2,000–2,499	2,500
Healthy infant	10	13	15	17	18	20
High-risk infant	10	10	13	15	17	18

Data from ref. 11.

Table 15-6. Narrowing down and management of neonatal jaundice

Cause	Type of bilirubin	Time of onset of jaundice (days)	Peak bilirubin		Management
			mg/dl	Age (days)	
Physiologic					
Full-term infant	Unconjugated	2–3	10–12	3	Reassurance
Premature infant	Unconjugated	3–4	15	9	Reassurance
Sepsis	Both	At any time	Rises more than 5 mg/ 24 hours		Cultures, blood group, Coombs test,
Blood group problem	Both	In 1st day	May be quite high		blood smear, consultation
Hyperbilirubinemia of newborn, cause usually unknown					
Full-term infant	Unconjugated	2–3	Greater than 12	1st week	Ensure that there is no blood group incompatibility
Premature infant	Unconjugated	3–4	Greater than 15	1st week	Phototherapy (Table 15-5); if unsatisfactory response, seek consultation

ever, there is NO CLEAR EVIDENCE that brain damage does not occur with lower levels of hyperbilirubinemia, since no long-term prospective studies have been conducted. The etiology for breast-milk jaundice is controversial, but one suggestion is that human breast milk contains large quantities of unsaturated fatty acids that inhibit hepatic bilirubin conjugation. Initial treatment includes phototherapy, and, in severe cases of an early, rapid rise of bilirubin, exchange transfusions may be necessary. Table 15-5 lists the guidelines for the use of phototherapy during the newborn period based on the differentiation of physiologic from nonphysiologic jaundice. Table 15-6 outlines the narrowing down and management of neonatal jaundice.

REFERENCES

1. Carderol, B., Hon, E. Neonatal bradycardia following nasopharyngeal stimulation. *J. Physiol.* 78:441–446, 1971.

2. Brown, W., Ostheimer, G., Bell, G., Datta, S.S. Newborn response to O_2 blown over the face. *Anesthesiology* 44:535–536, 1976.

3. Carson, B., Losey, B., Bowers, W., Simmons, M.A. Combined obstetric and pediatric approach to prevent meconium aspiration syndrome. *Am. J. Obstet. Gynecol.* 126:712–717, 1976.

4. Caspi, P., Ronin, J., Goldberg, L., Avery, M.E., Hehre, A., Fromm, B., Lawson, E., Neff, R.U. Prevention of respiratory distress syndrome in premature infants by ante-partum, gluco-cortocoid therapy. *Br. J. Obstet. Gynecol.* 83:967–973, 1976.

5. Taeusch, H., Jr., Frigoletto, F., Kitzmiller, J., Avery, M.E., Hehre, A., Fromm, B., Lawson, E., Neff, R.K. Risk of respiratory distress syndrome after pre-natal dexamethasone treatment. *Pediatrics* 63:64–72, 1979.

6. Carter, C.O. Congenital defects: The genetics of congenital malformations. *Proc. R. Soc. Med.* 61:991–997, 1968.

7. Sadounick, A., Baird, P. Incidence of neural tube defects in live-born and still-born infants in British Columbia over a 10-year period. *Can. Med. Assoc. J.* 129:1109–1110, 1983.

8. Owens, J. Letter. Recurrence rates of neural tube defects. *Lancet* 1:8440:1282, 1985.

9. Apgar, V. A proposal for a new method of evaluation of the newborn infant. *Analg.* 32:260, 1983.

10. Fyler, D.C. Report of the New England Regional Infant Cardiac Program. *Pediatrics* 65(suppl.):375–461, 1980.

11. Gartner, L.M. In *Haematology of Infancy and Childhood*, 2d ed., Nathan, D.G., Oski, F.A., eds. Philadelphia: W.B. Saunders, 1981, p. 105.

16

CONTROVERSIES IN CHILDHOOD NUTRITION

Comprehensive pediatric textbooks (1–3) contain excellent descriptions of the nutrient requirements of children in different age groups. The practicing physician, however, faces many questions not so easily answered by the standard texts. Health-conscious parents are bombarded daily with dogmatic statements in the media pertaining to the nutrition of infants and children. In this chapter, the ten major questions and controversies pertaining to childhood nutrition are discussed. Whenever possible, the evidence in support of or against various recommendations is provided. Table 16-1 lists the major controversies addressed.

CONTROVERSY NUMBER 1: ARE BOTTLE-FED BABIES AT RISK OF MEDICAL OR EMOTIONAL PROBLEMS?

Jelliffe and Jelliffe (4) suggest that bottle-fed babies are at risk of medical or emotional problems. Certainly, in developing countries where refrigeration, clean water, and adequate nutrition are often lacking, the risks are real. The question is whether the risks are present in the developed world. The Jelliffes list inadequacies in the nutritional components of artificial milk and describe studies that demonstrate breast-feeding to be superior in protecting the infant against infection, allergy, child abuse, and later psychosocial maladjustment.

Before one makes a recommendation to a pregnant woman about how to feed her infant, one should examine the quality of evidence upon which papers such as the Jelliffes' are based. Recently, the U.S. Department of Health and Human Services commissioned a task force "to examine the scientific evidence regarding infant-feeding and infant health in both the United States and developing countries"(5). The task force was given specific criteria by which to judge the evidence, including the strength of the association between type of feeding and infant health, whether confounding factors were

Table 16-1. Controversies in childhood nutrition

1. Breast- versus bottle-feeding of infants
2. Age to start solid foods
3. Are supplemental iron, fluorides, or vitamins needed?
4. Do infant formulas need to be sterilized?
5. Are fast foods really junk?
6. Is a vegetarian diet safe for children?
7. The role of dietary fiber
8. Food allergies—do they exist?
9. Food additives, behavior, and learning
10. Is atherosclerosis a pediatric problem?

accounted for, and what the effect of uncontrolled biases were likely to be. Their conclusion was that any health benefits that breast-feeding might confer, given a population with good sanitation, nutrition, and medical care, are "apparently modest." The "lack of firm evidence for an association between infant health and feeding practice is due to poor study design; in only a few studies were confounding factors controlled." Using similar criteria, the authors reviewed the evidence that "breast feeding protects against later psychological maladjustment" and came to a similar conclusion: Given the poor quality of the evidence, one can state that there are no grounds for ascribing an improved psychological outcome in the child to either breast- or bottle-feeding (6).

Infants who nurse well or who take prepared infant formula, and who are shown love, attention, and stimulation, will do well both physically and mentally.

Breast-feeding is enjoying a revival in the developed world. Certainly for mothers who wish to and are financially able to remain at home and for whom nursing comes easily, this form of infant nutrition is the most convenient and low-cost. Although there are real advantages, problems develop when doctors and nurses become evangelical about breast-feeding and put great pressure on mothers who do not wish to nurse or who cannot.

CONTROVERSY NUMBER 2: SHOULD INFANTS START SOLID FOODS EARLY (1 MONTH) OR LATE (AFTER 4 MONTHS)?

As with the controversy regarding breast- versus bottle-feeding, many dogmatic statements have been made on the basis of very flimsy evidence. There is NO CLEAR EVIDENCE that infants need solid foods before 4 to 6 months. The major additional nutrient required at around this age is iron, and the major source of iron is infant cereal. There is NO CLEAR EVIDENCE that the early introduction of solids helps infants sleep through the night. There is also NO CLEAR EVIDENCE that the introduction of solids earlier is harmful.

The current consensus is that infant cereals should be started at 4 to 6 months because they contain iron.

CONTROVERSY NUMBER 3: ARE SUPPLEMENTAL IRON, FLUORIDES, OR VITAMINS NEEDED?

Although iron supplementation has been recommended (7), in the form of either iron drops or iron-fortified milk formula, there is SUGGESTIVE EVIDENCE that this is not necessary for the majority of full-term infants who are otherwise healthy (8). Breast-fed and formula-fed infants started on infant cereals at 4 to 6 months need neither iron drops nor iron-fortified milk. Although the ingestion of fluoride is clearly related to better teeth, there is NO CLEAR EVIDENCE that fluoride supplements are beneficial before the teeth erupt. There is little fluoride in breast milk. Infants whose formula is reconstituted with fluoridated water do not need additional fluoride. Family physicians should inquire of local health authorities as to the fluoride content of the local water supply; if it is less than 0.3 parts per million, supplemental fluoride in the form of sodium fluoride drops is recommended.

Infants fed commercial formulas do not need supplemental vitamins. Since human milk contains little vitamin D (9), 400 IU of vitamin D has been recommended for breast-fed babies; however, rickets in wholly breast-fed infants is seen only in the offspring of mothers with inadequate vitamin D stores who maintain a strict vegan vegetarian diet and who receive little exposure to sunlight.

Formula-fed infants need no additional vitamin C, since commercially available infant formulas already contain vitamin C. Human milk contains adequate amounts of vitamin C.

Once infants reach 6 months of age, they no longer need to drink prepared infant formula; they can take whole cow's milk. There is SUGGESTIVE EVIDENCE that whole milk is preferable to 2% milk for infants. Commercially available cow's milk has adequate vitamin D added. By this age, infants will most likely be taking fruit juices, which will provide adequate vitamin C. Thus, supplemental vitamins and iron are rarely needed for the healthy infant eating adequate amounts of milk, cereal, and fruit juices. After infancy, children who eat a balanced Western diet do not need supplemental vitamins.

CONTROVERSY NUMBER 4: DO INFANT FORMULAS NEED TO BE STERILIZED?

Although a leading pediatric text recommends sterilizing bottles, equipment, and formula (3), it is clear that this recommendation is no longer valid (10) (FIRM EVIDENCE). Careful washing of the hands, bottles, and bottle nipples, and refrigeration of the prepared formula, are all that is necessary.

CONTROVERSY NUMBER 5: ARE FAST FOODS REALLY JUNK?

Many physicians and parents confuse the two terms, "fast food" and "junk food." Junk foods are defined as those foods that have no nutritional value other than providing calories (11). Fast foods are those prepared quickly in fast-food outlets.

Adolescents (and almost everyone else) enjoy both junk foods and fast foods. Although too much junk food may increase obesity or diminish the appetite for more nutritional foods, fast foods are not necessarily junk and should not be proscribed. In fact, analysis of some of the more popular fast foods shows that they are quite nutritious and, if consumed judiciously as part of a well-balanced diet, are perfectly acceptable (11). An example of fast food is pizza, which is quite nutritious, whereas an example of junk food is a jelly donut, which consists mainly of empty calories.

CONTROVERSY NUMBER 6: IS A VEGETARIAN DIET SAFE FOR CHILDREN?

Some parents who are vegetarians insist on rearing their infants as vegetarians. Some authorities recommend against this practice (12). For mothers who are willing to breast-feed their infants and who themselves have an adequate intake of vitamins, proteins, and minerals, there should be no problems, as least as long as the infants are breast-feeding. For vegetarians who do not breast-feed, a commercial soy-based formula is satisfactory, as long as the infant starts eating iron-enriched cereals by 4 to 6 months of age. Between 6 and 12 months, vegetables, fruit, pureed legumes, tofu, and nut butters should be added to the diet. When the infant discontinues commercial soy-milk formula, supplemental vitamin D should be given until 2 years of age. In those families whose only proscription is animal meat but who do eat milk and eggs, a balanced diet is much easier to achieve. Given careful attention to nutrition, a completely vegetable diet can be safe; when poor nutrition occurs, it is due more to an insufficient quantity of food than to the choice of foods (13,14).

CONTROVERSY NUMBER 7: WHAT IS THE ROLE OF DIETARY FIBER?

Lack of dietary fiber has been linked to constipation, bowel cancer, coronary heart disease, irritable bowel syndrome, and diverticulitis. Whereas fiber and its role in health and disease have been studied in adults, the exact role of dietary fiber in children's health is largely unknown. In spite of this, an increased intake of dietary fiber is being widely promoted by the media. The amount and nature of the fiber ingested by the average infant and child in the developed world are not known. There is FIRM EVIDENCE that adding fiber to the diet of children with idiopathic recurrent abdominal pain is beneficial (15) (see Chapter 22). At present, there is NO CLEAR EVIDENCE that more fiber than that provided in a properly balanced diet containing fruit, cereals, and vegetables is required for the average child (16).

CONTROVERSY NUMBER 8: FOOD ALLERGIES— DO THEY EXIST?

Food allergies have been incriminated in many problems of infancy and childhood. Allergy to cow's milk is thought by many to cause colic. A cohort study at Yale University showed no differences in the incidence of colic in babies fed either human or cow's milk. Confounding variables were controlled by stepwise logistic regression (17) (SUGGESTIVE EVIDENCE).

For many years, cow's milk and the early introduction of solid foods were thought to be causally related to atopic eczema and other allergic conditions. A recent case-control study that controlled for confounding variables and in which the observers were blinded concluded that "breast feeding and delayed introduction of solids do not protect against atopic eczema" (18) (SUGGESTIVE EVIDENCE). However, one cannot generalize: A recent double-blind, randomized, controlled trial of dietary treatments found that children with migraine had symptoms when certain foods were added to the diet, especially milk, eggs, and chocolate (19) (FIRM EVIDENCE). However the sample was not typical of children with migraine.

Probably the most logical approach in this controversy is to be aware that, for most conditions and for most children, it is unlikely that foods cause the problem symptoms. For some children and for some conditions (e.g., migraine), it may well be that foods are contributing factors. Instead of advising complicated rotating diets or oligoantigenic diets, the physician should listen to the parents' observations. If certain foods regularly appear to cause symptoms, and if these foods are not nutritionally required or can be substituted for, a trial of withholding and reintroducing them may be worthwhile.

CONTROVERSY NUMBER 9: DO FOOD ADDITIVES HAVE A DELETERIOUS EFFECT ON BEHAVIOR AND LEARNING?

In 1974, Feingold published a book for parents that received international attention (20). The reason for the book's popularity was that a complex and difficult problem—childhood hyperactivity—was reduced to a simple model: certain foods such as apples, citrus fruits, and tomatoes cause hyperactivity, and, in addition, all food additives are also causative. Thus if a hyperactive child did not improve on Dr. Feingold's diet, it was because either the child was cheating or the parents were not sufficiently careful. Unfortunately, the problem of childhood hyperactivity is not so simple. In a randomized, double-blind, crossover trial, the Feingold diet was found to be ineffective (21) (FIRM EVIDENCE). As with the controversy involving food allergies, however, the physician's policy should not be rigid. If parents claim that a specific food or food additive regularly affects their child's behavior adversely, and if that food substance is not essential or can be substituted for, the parent's view can be supported.

CONTROVERSY NUMBER 10: IS ATHEROSCLEROSIS A PEDIATRIC PROBLEM?

Autopsies have shown evidence of atherosclerosis even in young soldiers killed in battle. This has led some to suggest that physicians who look after infants and children should play a role in preventing coronary heart disease and strokes. By advocating the start of a diet low in animal fat in infancy, it is postulated that atherosclerosis-related morbidity and mortality can be prevented in adult life. In one prospective study, ninety-five infants were followed for 4 years (22). There was no correlation between the type and duration of early infant feeding and subsequent serum lipid levels. By the age of 3 to 4 years, the serum cholesterol concentration correlated with that of the parents. The definitive answer to this controversy can be established only by a prospective randomized, controlled trial from infancy to old age: Clearly, such a study will never be done. For the moment, it might be more prudent to do research on the lipid levels of infants and children with strong family histories of early coronary heart disease, to see if abnormal levels could be lowered. Such a study has not yet been done. Western society has become much more conscious about the possible relationship between diet and coronary heart disease. It is likely that changes in the dietary habits of adults will have an effect on the diets of infants and children as well.

In nutrition, as in other aspects of health care, it is important to be aware of the quality of the evidence supporting certain recommendations. When good evidence is not available, family physicians should not jump on the latest nutrition bandwagon; they should take care to give reasonable dietary advice to parents.

REFERENCES

1. *Current Pediatric Diagnosis and Treatment*, 8th ed., Kempe, C.H., Silver, H.K, O'Brien, D., eds. Los Altos, Calif.: Lange Medical Publications, 1984.

2. *Pediatrics*, 17th ed., Rudolph, A.M., Hoffman, J.E., Axebrod, S., eds. Norwalk, Conn.: Appleton-Centry-Crofts, 1982.
3. *Nelson Textbook of Pediatrics*, 12th ed., Behrman, R.E., Vaughan, V.C., eds. Philadelphia: W.B. Saunders, 1983.
4. Jelliffe, D.B., Jelliffe, E.F.P. Current concepts in nutrition. "Breast is best": Modern meanings. *N. Engl. J. Med.* 297:912–915, 1977.
5. Report of the Task Force on the Assessment of the Scientific Evidence Relating to Infant-Feeding Practices and Infant Health. *Pediatrics* 74(4)(suppl.):579–762, 1984.
6. Feldman, W., Hodgson, C., Goodman, J., Turgay, A. Breast-feeding and psychological benefit to children: The quality of the evidence. *Clin. Invest. Med.* 8:A182 (Abstract), 1985.
7. *Nelson Textbook of Pediatrics*, 12th ed., Behrman, R.E., Vaughan, V.C., eds. Nutrition and Nutritional Disorders. Philadelphia: W.B. Saunders, 1983.
8. Feldman, W., Greene-Finestone, L., Heick, H., Luke, B. Do all infants need to be screened for anemia or iron deficiency? *Clin. Invest. Med.* 8:3, A182 (Abstract), 1985.
9. Greer, F.R., Reeve, L.E., Chesney, R.W., DeLuca, H.F. Water-soluble vitamin D in human milk: A myth. *Pediatrics* 69:238, 1982.
10. Gerber, M.A., Berliner, B.C., Karolus, J.J. Sterilization of infant formula. *Clin. Pediatr.* 22:344–349, 1983.
11. Zlotkin, S.H. Controversies in nutrition, 1984. *Modern Medicine of Canada* 39:443–448, 1984.
12. Nutrition Committee of the Canadian Pediatric Society. Infant feeding practices revisited. *Can. Med. Assoc. J.* 122:987–989, 1980.
13. Shinwell, E.D. Totally vegetarian diets and infant nutrition. *Pediatrics* 70:582–586, 1982.
14. Christoffel, K. A pediatric perspective on vegetarian nutrition. *Clin. Pediatr.* 20:632–643, 1981.
15. Feldman, W., McGrath, P., Hodgson, C., Ritter, H., Shipman, R.T. The use of dietary fiber in the management of simple childhood idiopathic recurrent abdominal pain: Results in a prospective double-blind randomized controlled trial. *Am. J. Dis. Child.* 139:1216–1218, 1985.
16. Report from the Committee on Nutrition, Massachussetts Medical Society. *N. Engl. J. Med.* 304:1102–1104, 1981.
17. Forsyth, B.W.C., Leventhal, J.M., McCarthy, P.L. Mothers' perceptions of problems of feeding and crying behaviours. *Am. J. Dis. Child.* 139:269–272, 1985.
18. Kramer, M.S., Moroz, B. Do breast-feeding and delayed introduction of solid foods protect against subsequent atopic eczema? *J. Pediatr.* 98:546–550, 1981.
19. Egger, J., Wilson, J., Carter, C.M., Turner, M.W., Soothill, J.F. Is migraine a food allergy? *Lancet* 2:865–869, 1983.
20. Feingold, B.F.F. *Why Your Child Is Hyperactive*. New York: Random House, 1974.
21. Harley, J.P., Mathews, C.G. The Feingold hypothesis: Current studies. *Modern Medicine of Canada* 33:1219–1222, 1978.
22. Anderson, G.E., Lipschitz, C., Friis-Hansen, B. Dietary habits and serum lipids during the first 4 years of life. *Acta Paediatr. Scand.* 68:165–170, 1979.

17

PROBLEMS OF EATING

Problems of eating include obesity; anorexia and bulimia; the consumption of nonfood substances (pica); dental problems; and food choices and behavior at mealtimes. Problems of growth are treated in Chapter 19. Issues of breast-feeding are described in Chapter 16. Accidental poisoning is covered in Chapter 24.

PREVALENCE

The prevalence of obesity depends on the definition of the condition. The most common definition is weight above the eightieth percentile for the height, age, and sex of the child. This definition results in a 20% incidence of obesity in children. With other definitions, obesity has been estimated to occur in between 3 and 40% of children (1).

The prevalence of clinical anorexia has been conservatively estimated to be 1 in 250 in girls under 16 and 1 in 100 in girls over age 16 (2). However, approximately 50% of adolescent girls but only 20% of adolescent boys believe themselves to be overweight and want to lose weight even if they are of normal weight (3). The prevalence of clinical bulimia is unknown, but bulimic behavior (i.e., out-of-control binging) is reported to occur in one-third of adolescent girls and one-sixth of adolescent boys (3). There is a widespread belief and some evidence (4) that the prevalence of both disorders is increasing. The prevalence of clinical anorexia and bulimia is 7.6% in high-risk groups such as highly competitive female dancers (4).

Pica is common in children up to 1 year old but rare in the normal population above that age (5). However, pica occurs in between 8 and 28% of older mentally retarded children and adults. Complications of pica include lead poisoning, intestinal obstruction, constipation, and nutritional anemia.

By the age of 11 the average American child has three decayed permanent teeth, and the average 17-year-old has eight to nine decayed, filled, or missing teeth (6). Untreated tooth decay is a major health problem in children over

5 years old. Periodontal disease frequently begins in childhood and has been estimated to affect half the children in the world (7).

Problems with food choices and behavior at mealtimes are common. Between 6 and 40% of preschool-aged children are estimated to have feeding problems (8), but often no distinction is made between food choices and behavior problems at mealtimes.

OBESITY

Narrowing down

Narrowing down the problem of obesity is complicated by the extreme difficulty of deciding the criteria for obesity and the strong belief held by many normal-weight adolescents (especially girls) that they are overweight (3). However, for the primary care physician, obesity can be defined as a child's weighing more than 20% above his or her appropriate weight for height, using standard growth charts. There are exceptions to this "rule of thumb." Children who are very muscular may not be obese and yet be overweight. Children who are very unfit may be of normal weight but obese.

Management of obesity

The management of obesity is a major industry in the Western world. Medicine can intervene both in the prevention of obesity and in its treatment. Kramer et al. (9) found SUGGESTIVE EVIDENCE that breast-feeding may result in less obesity at age 2. However, the size of the difference between the weights of breast-fed and formula-fed infants is small. For example, every 10 weeks of exclusive breast-feeding led to a 244-g lessening in weight or a 0.566-mm difference in skin-fold summed from three locations. Birth weight and maternal weight were also significant factors in the child's weight at 2 years. Piscano et al. (10) found that the Prudent Diet prescribed to infants at 3 months of age resulted in significantly fewer obese children at 3 years of age; this can be regarded as SUGGESTIVE EVIDENCE of the efficacy of preventive procedures. The efficacy of primary care interventions for childhood obesity once obesity has developed has not been demonstrated.

The physician faced with an obese pediatric patient should counsel moderation and a sensible diet combined with moderate exercise. This type of program has been shown to be effective in reducing weight and increasing fitness (11) (FIRM EVIDENCE) when delivered in a structured, intensive 10-week program with monthly follow-up involving both the child and the parents. The efficacy of such a program in primary care has not been assessed but is likely to be limited unless a comprehensive structured program is initiated. Referral to a consultant (dietician, psychologist, or clinic) experienced in this type of management of obesity in children may be appropriate.

Although there is NO CLEAR EVIDENCE for the following guidelines for dealing with an obese child, they are based on clinical experience and related literature (12). These guidelines are appropriate for children over 5 years of age.

1. See the parents and child separately.
2. Teach parents to praise the child for progress in weight loss *and* exercise.
3. Have the child and/or parents keep detailed diaries of food intake *and* exercise.
4. Clearly specify the goals of weight loss (e.g., 1–3 pounds) per week and exercise (3–4 miles of walking per day or equivalent) in a written agreement. An organized exercise program is preferred, especially for the first few months.
5. Keep in mind that, in the case of a younger child, the goal may be to maintain a constant weight, since linear growth will represent weight loss.
6. Prescribe and ensure that a nutritionally adequate diet is followed. Monitor height to determine if it tracks with expected growth.
7. Ensure that inappropriate foods such as candy and other high-calorie snacks are not in the home.
8. Be prepared for a long-term program that will take several months of intensive work and years of follow-up.
9. Avoid power struggles between parents and child and between physician and child.

Perhaps most important, the child should be encouraged to perceive the doctor as a source of information and support. If other family members over-eat and under-exercise, the prognosis for weight loss and fitness in the child is not good. If the whole family is committed to a sensible diet and exercise, the child is more likely to benefit. The major negative outcomes of childhood obesity may well be the social isolation, self-hatred, and poor physical fitness that are often its concomitants. Unrealistic expectations on the part of the physician may increase feelings of guilt and self-hatred in the child.

ANOREXIA AND BULIMIA

Narrowing down

Anorexia nervosa consists of a constellation of symptoms that include (a) an intense, unremitting fear of being fat; (b) a feeling of being fat even when emaciated; (c) weight loss of 25% body weight at the beginning of the disorder, plus the weight gain that could be expected on the basis of growth charts; (d) refusal to maintain weight over a minimal weight for age and height; and (e) no physical illness that would account for such weight loss (13).

Bulimia is binge eating in which high-calorie food is eaten, often secretly, until the person is prevented from further eating by abdominal pain, sleep, interruption, or vomiting. There are often weight fluctuations resulting from the alternation of binges and periods of fasting, vomiting, or use of cathartics or diuretics. The bulimic knows the pattern is abnormal, fears being unable to stop eating, and feels depressed after binges (13). Bulimics are often of normal weight.

The patients usually are brought to the attention of a physician because of parents' concern about restrictive diets or induced vomiting. Children and adolescents who ask their doctors about dieting or who express concern about being fat (when they are not) should be queried further. Adolescent females as a group should be considered at risk for anorexic and bulimic behaviors and should be given the opportunity to discuss these issues. A two-step strategy can be used: All adolescent girls can be asked how they feel about their weight. Those that are concerned can be asked about binges and the use of laxatives, diuretics, or vomiting. Questions such as, "Some adolescents who are worried about their weight make themselves sick or use laxatives to lose weight. Do you?" are usually accepted by teenagers. Any dramatic reduction in weight or the cessation of menstrual periods should raise the physician's suspicions. The *Diagnostic and Statistical Manual of Mental Disorders* of the American Psychiatric Association (13) considers anorexia nervosa and bulimia to be separate disorders; however, the two often coexist.

Management of anorexia and bulimia

Management of clinical anorexia nervosa and bulimia includes referral of the patient to a consultant—in some cases, hospitalization—and almost certainly long-term therapy (14). Management of the rather more widespread subclinical syndromes that do not meet the criteria for formal diagnosis depends on the severity of the disorder. Although there is NO CLEAR EVIDENCE that early intervention is effective, the following guidelines are offered from clinical experience:

1. Schedule an appointment to discuss the issue with the adolescent privately.
2. Determine what situations or thoughts trigger eating restriction, binging, or purging.
3. Detail the medical and other consequences of the behavior, for example, dental damage, facial hair growth, or hospitalization with no ward privileges for nonattainment of weight goals may be an important incentive to encourage weight gain.
4. Assist the adolescent with problem solving. How can she avoid the situation that triggers the response or control the urges? How realistic are the thoughts that contribute to the problem? What alternatives are available?

5. Meet with the parents to encourage their helpful behavior, such as not urging a child with anorexic tendencies to eat very high calorie foods such as chocolate bars and encouraging regular, well-balanced meals.
6. Follow-up on a weekly basis. If the child's weight does not increase or continues to decrease, an urgent consultation is required.

There is evidence that adolescents are eager to talk to their physicians about these issues (15).

EATING OF NONFOOD SUBSTANCES (PICA)

Pica is the repetitive eating of nonfood substances past the first year of life.

Management of pica

Pica is managed by treating any acute symptoms and reducing the availability of nonfood substances by changing the environment (such as not letting the child play on dirt surfaces) and by increasing supervision and appropriate stimulation. Referral to a consultant is appropriate if pica continues.

DENTAL PROBLEMS

Narrowing down

Dental problems can be narrowed down by visual inspection of the teeth and gums, by asking parents about what is being fed the child, asking about frequency of tooth-brushing and flossing, and inquiring about dental visits.

Management of dental problems

Prevention of dental caries in nursing infants depends on the parents' not giving their infant a bottle of milk, juice, or sweetened drink at bedtime (15). Primary care physicians are best able to advise parents, since most children will not be seen by a dentist until after the damage is done. The frequency of sugar intake appears to be more important than the absolute amount of sugar intake. Consequently, snacking on sugar-laden, sticky foods should be discouraged. Physicians should encourage early visits (by 2½ years of age) to a dentist for dental education and to prevent fear of the dentist. Fluoridation of community water supplies and topical application of fluorides are effective in preventing decay (7) (FIRM EVIDENCE). Administration of supplemental fluorides is indicated where the water supply is not fluoridated. There is FIRM EVIDENCE that brushing and flossing can prevent periodontal disease (7). These practices should be strongly promoted by the family physician, but there is NO CLEAR EVIDENCE such encouragement is effective.

FOOD CHOICES AND BEHAVIOR AT MEALTIMES

Narrowing down

The parents should be questioned about their child's problems at mealtimes and asked to describe in detail what happens. The physician must then distinguish parental overconcern from actual problems. The key issue is how much the behavior disrupts the family. For example, a 3-year-old's invariant breakfast cereal preference and refusal of eggs and toast should not be a source of concern and can easily be accommodated. On the other hand, if the same child throws his food on the floor or demands a different meal than what has already been prepared, there is a problem.

Management of food choices and behavior at mealtimes

Restricted food choices or picky eating is best approached by very minimal intervention: encouragement of a variety of gradual changes in the range of foods eaten and avoidance of a power struggle that cannot be won. On the one hand, a child's right to prefer some foods should be balanced against the parents' right to expect that a special diet not be prepared for each member of the family. Parents should be discouraged from using punishment and emotional confrontation and encouraged to use praise and other forms of positive reinforcement for small changes in behavior. The parents' appropriate eating habits and behaviors, the availability of a range of foods, and the maintenance of a pleasant atmosphere at mealtimes will usually produce results. Parental anxiety is real and should be met with sincere discussion focusing on the wide range of normal behaviors. Demonstrating, with the use of growth charts, that the child is growing normally will often allay parents' fears that their child is not eating enough. Frequently, parents do not know how much food a child should eat or that most children are picky eaters at one time or another.

Management of problem behaviors at mealtime in the home consists of ignoring minor misbehavior, praising appropriate behavior, and removing the child to a boring place for 2 to 5 minutes ("time out") for major disruptive behavior. There is FIRM EVIDENCE that this program, in the form of a simple written protocol given to the parents, can be effective (16).

Behavior problems that occur when children eat out with their parents are particularly trying for many families. There is FIRM EVIDENCE that when parents follow a series of specific suggestions, improved behavior results:

1. Tell the child exactly what is expected of him or her at the restaurant.
2. Find a table or booth away from the crowd.
3. Seat the child on the inside, next to the wall.
4. Separate the children, if there is more than one in the family.
5. Provide the child with a premeal snack, such as crackers.
6. Order food that the child will enjoy.

7. Provide small interesting toys to occupy the child until the food comes.
8. Move utensils out of the child's reach.
9. Remove the toys when food arrives.
10. Periodically praise the child for appropriate behavior.

Concern about eating behavior in a child less than 18 months should be regarded as evidence of the parents' unrealistic expectations and should trigger further inquiry about other "misbehavior." Guidance and close follow-up is required, as the child may be at risk for abuse.

REFERENCES

1. Stunkard, A.J., d'Aquili, E., Fox, S., Filion, R.D.L. Influence of social class on obesity and thinness in children. *J. Am. Med Assoc.* 221:579–584, 1972.
2. Crisp, A.H., Palmer, R.L., Kalucy, R.S. How common is anorexia nervosa? A prevalence study. *Br. J. Psychiatry* 128:549–554, 1976.
3. Feldman, W., McGrath, P., O'Shaughnesy, M. Adolescents' pursuit of thinness. *Am. J. Dis. Child.* 140:294, 1986.
4. Frankenberg, F., Garfinkel, P.E., Garner, D.M. Anorexia nervosa: Issues in prevention. *Journal of Preventive Psychiatry* 1:469–483, 1982.
5. Baltrop, D. The prevalence of pica. *Am. J. Dis. Child.* 112:116–123, 1966.
6. U.S. Department of Health and Human Services. *Better Health for Our Children: A National Strategy,* vol. 1. Report of the Select Panel for the Promotion of Child Health. Washington: U.S. Government Printing Office, 1981.
7. Leske, G.S., Ripa, L.W., Leske, M.C. Dental public health. In *Public Health and Preventive Medicine,* 11th ed., Last, J., ed. New York: Appleton-Century-Crofts, 1980.
8. Hertzler, A.A. Children's food patterns—A review: 1. Food preferences and feeding problems. *J. Am. Diet. Assoc.* 83:551–554, 1983.
9. Kramer, M.S., Barr, R.G., Leduc, D.G., Boisjoly, C., Pless, I.B. Infant determinants of childhood weight and adiposity. *J. Pediatr.* 107:104–107, 1985.
10. Piscano, J.C., Lichter, H., Ritter, J., Siegal, A.P. An attempt at prevention of obesity in infancy. *Pediatrics* 61:360–364, 1978.
11. Epstein, L.H., Wing, R.R., Penner, B.C., Kress, M.J. Effect of diet and controlled exercise on weight loss in obese children. *J. Pediatr.* 107:358–61, 1985.
12. Epstein, L.H., Wing, R.R., Valoski, A. Childhood obesity. *Pediatr. Clin. North Am.* 32:363–379, 1985.
13. American Psychiatric Association. *Diagnostic and Statistical Manual of Mental Disorders,* 3d ed. Washington, D.C.: American Psychiatric Association, 1980.
14. Garfinkel, P.E., Garner, D.M. *Anorexia Nervosa: A Multidimensional Perspective.* New York: Brunner/Mazel, 1982.
15. Hodgson, C., Feldman, W., Corber, S., Quinn, A. Adolescent health needs: II. Utilization of health care by adolescents. *Adolescence* 21:383–390, 1986.
16. Snawder, K. The nursing-bottle syndrome and related problems. In *Current Therapy in Dentistry,* vol. 5, Goldman, H.M., Gilmore, H.W., Irby, W.B., Olsen, N.H., eds. St. Louis: C.V. Mosby, 1974.

17. McMahon, R.J., Forehand, R. Non-prescriptive behavior therapy: Effectiveness of a brochure in teaching mothers to correct their children's inappropriate meal-time behaviors. *Behav. Ther.* 9:814–820, 1978.
18. Bauman, K.E., Reiss, M., Rogers, R.W., Bailey, J.S. Dining out with children: Effectiveness of a parent advice package on pre-meal inappropriate behavior. *J. Appl. Behav. Anal.* 16:55–68, 1983.

18

PROBLEMS OF SLEEPING

Problems of sleeping in children and adolescents are commonly mentioned by parents who consult with primary care physicians. They can be divided into four categories (1): falling asleep and waking up during the night; excessive sleepiness; problems with the sleep-wake schedule; and episodic events during sleep, including bed-wetting (see Chapter 10), sleepwalking, sleeptalking, nightmares, night terrors, head-banging, and teeth-grinding.

PREVALENCE

"Normal" sleep patterns in infancy have not been firmly established, but it is known that between 25 and 50% of children under 1 year of age have difficulties sleeping through the night (2–4). Problems in falling asleep, as reported by parents, have been estimated to occur in approximately 20% of 2- to 5-year-olds (5), and waking at night has been reported in close to 40% of 2- to 5-year-olds (5). Problems in falling asleep in school-aged children (5 to 12 years old) appear to be less frequent than in toddlers but may be of greater severity. Almost 40% of adolescents report occasional difficulties in falling asleep and maintaining sleep, while 13% report chronic severe problems (6).

The prevalence of excessive sleepiness in infants and young children is not known, but it is a relatively rare complaint. Although the frequency of sleepiness in school-aged children and adolescents has not been well documented, it is usually seen as a problem only when it interferes with school activities. The prevalence of narcolepsy in children is about 1 in 1,200 (3). The prevalence of apnea-hypersomnia syndrome in children is unknown but the condition is rare.

The prevalence of problems with the sleep-wake schedule in children is unknown. Nor is the prevalence of parasomnias (episodic events during sleep) known.

FALLING ASLEEP AND WAKING DURING THE NIGHT

Narrowing down and diagnosis

Narrowing down the problem of falling asleep and waking during the night requires parental reports for infants, toddlers, and school-aged children, and self-reports and parental reports for adolescents. Polysomnographic recording is very rarely required. Difficulties in falling asleep and waking may be developmentally normal; secondary to drug or alcohol use; the result of physical illness; due to behavior problems, anxiety, or depression; a response to the parents' marital problems; or due to other sleep disorders, such as apnea or narcolepsy. Table 18-1 summarizes the indications and management of each problem.

Problems in falling asleep or in waking occur at all ages but are most marked in infancy: this phenomenon is so common that it may be a normal developmental phase. Some children have disturbed sleep in infancy and continue to have irregular sleep patterns (5); this is not pathological and has been correlated with a temperament characterized by a low sensory threshold (7), with demand breast-feeding and sleeping in the same room as the parents (8), and with obstetrical problems (9). The early onset and persistence of the problem are the clearest indications of a normal developmental variation. Some children with this normal pattern learn that crying and not falling asleep will get them considerable attention from their parents. Many

Table 18-1. Problems in falling asleep and waking too early in children

Type	Age	Narrowing down	Management
Normal	All ages	Early onset, low sensory threshold	Reduce sensory input; behavior management
Drug- or alcohol-induced	All ages	Use of drugs or alcohol	Discontinue use of drugs or alcohol
Behavior problem	Over 6 months	Situational crying; in older children, other compliance problems	Behavior management
Anxiety	Over 4 years	Ruminations, fears in bed	Treat anxiety
Depression	Over 4 years	Depressed mood, other depressive features	Treat depression
Parents' marital problems	Any age	Parental disputes triggering stress and/or compliance problems	Treat marital problems
Apnea/ narcolepsy*			

*See Table 18-2.

such parents resent the excessive time they must spend with their child at bedtime.

A dependence on hypnotic drugs can develop within 1 week of use and has been reported to be a common cause of the severest forms of insomnia in infants (10). Alcohol can be ingested at any age and may cause waking at night. One should not assume that drugs or alcohol are not being consumed by children. Specific questions should be asked about what is being given to the child. One hundred milliliters of "gripe water," for example, contains 5 milliliters of 90-proof alcohol, and some over-the-counter cough and teething medicines also contain considerable amounts of alcohol.

Difficulty getting the child with behavior problems to go to and stay in bed is exceedingly common and may seriously disrupt the parent-child and marital relationships. Typically, the child either stalls going to bed or gets out of bed after having been put to bed. The parents will report repeated instances of this form of noncompliance.

Behavioral bedtime difficulties can be distinguished from anxiety-based bedtime difficulties by assessing how genuine are the fears that the child expresses. Children with behavior problems in going to bed usually express fears as an excuse for noncompliance with the bedtime. These anxieties are only an afterthought. Anxiety-based bedtime problems in children may be the result of some terrifying event or bad dreams. To find out what is worrying the child, it is best to interview both the child and the parents. Fear of physical or sexual abuse at any age and in both sexes must be considered. Direct questioning of the child in private with questions such as, "Are you afraid someone might hurt you?" or "Has anyone ever hurt you or scared you in bed?" is warranted.

A form of anxiety-type sleep-onset problem occurs in adolescence and is similar to adult insomnia. Teenagers report difficulty falling asleep and that they ruminate about their sleep problem and other worries. They frequently have poor "sleep hygiene"; they do many activities in bed, experience long periods of tossing and turning, and often have to nap to catch up on their sleep.

Sleep problems resulting from depression become more common as the child grows older and are accompanied by depressive mood and behavior. Difficulty falling asleep and early awakening are typical.

Sleep problems that are due to the parents' marital distress are often narrowed down by questions to the parents about the management of bedtime, "Do you and your spouse agree on how to handle the bedtime problem?" and by questions about frequency and timing of conflicts, "How often and when do you and your spouse argue, disagree, or fight?" or, "How is your marriage going?"

Some children may have multiple causes for their difficulties in falling asleep or waking in the night. Difficulty falling asleep or waking in the night that is not disruptive and is accompanied by the ability to fall asleep when ready does not present a problem and rarely is brought to the attention of the physician.

Management of falling asleep and maintaining sleep

The management of problems in falling asleep and maintaining sleep depends on their cause. Normal difficulties of falling asleep or maintaining sleep are best dealt with by reassurance that the pattern is normal and that it is impossible to force sleep. However, it is possible to enhance the probability of sleep by reducing sensory input and by not reinforcing crying that is designed to get attention.

Weissbluth (11) described a management program for crying problems that may have been learned when a child had colic. This regimen is appropriate for all infants over the age of 3 months who are having difficulty falling asleep. The program has four stages, each of which is carried out until the infant's sleep is reliably triggered: (a) soothing without picking the baby up, (b) reducing the extent of parental soothing responses, (c) limiting the time of parental soothing responses, (d) delaying the parental response. There is SUGGESTIVE EVIDENCE that this program is effective.

Children who have difficulty falling asleep or who wake at night should be expected to stay quietly in their beds and to look at a book or play quietly with a toy. Failure to comply with this expectation should be treated as a behavior problem (see below).

Drug- or alcohol-induced sleep problems are managed by withdrawal of the drug. Hypnotics should be withdrawn gradually. Sleep problems due to physical illness are managed by treatment of the underlying disorder. Chronic problems should not be treated with the chronic administration of hypnotics.

Sleep problems resulting from behavior disorders can often be readily managed by means of behavioral interventions. Behavioral protocols have been established that enable the health professional to teach parents how to deal with these behavior problems. The program consists of having the parents establish a "quiet time" for 30 minutes prior to a regularly established bedtime routine, such as a bedtime story, a drink of water or milk or juice, bathroom activities, and kisses and hugs. The child is put to bed, the light is turned out, and the parents leave. Crying, requests, or complaining are ignored. If the child gets out of bed, he or she is immediately returned to bed, with a single spank on the behind.[*] The child is rewarded with praise in the morning for compliance, a calendar with stars or stickers, and an activity reinforcer, such as being allowed to choose between two favorite foods for break-

---

[*]It is not clear that the spank is needed. Many families and many physicians find spanking unacceptable. Families that show the potential for child abuse should *never* be advised to spank their children.

fast. It is important to reassure the parent that crying will not hurt the child or cause the child any psychological damage.

The parents' persistence in this program is crucial, and they should not begin the program unless they are willing to see it through. Giving in to the child after beginning the program will make the behavior worse. The doctor or nurse should be available by phone to answer questions and provide support to the parents on the first few critical days of the program. There is FIRM EVIDENCE that this approach is effective (12–14).

Treatment of anxiety-based sleep problems requires, if possible, the removal of the cause of the anxiety. The management should then follow the program designed for behavioral problems. Care should be taken not to frighten the child; thus, a more gradual approach is advised. For example, for the child who refuses to go to bed because of a fear of the dark, use of a night-light combined with the parents initially sitting in the corner of the room should be the first step in a program designed to get the child to sleep alone in the room (NO CLEAR EVIDENCE).

Very brief (1 week or less) pharmacotherapy, using diphenhydramine, has been recommended for sleep difficulties (NO CLEAR EVIDENCE). The dosage for children under 6 years of age is 12.5 to 25 milligrams at bedtime. Older children may need from 25 to 100 milligrams at bedtime (15,16). A double-blind trial of trimeprazine tartrate in 1- and 2-year-olds with severe sleep problems did find statistically significant improvement, but it was clinically slight and not maintained (17).

Problems in falling asleep and waking in adolescents can be approached in the same way as those in adults. There is FIRM EVIDENCE that both relaxation training and stimulus control procedures are efficacious in reducing sleep onset latencies (18) in adults, but these techniques have not been evaluated in adolescents. Stimulus control instructions have the advantages of simplicity of use and superiority of effect. Following are stimulus control instructions adapted for adolescents:

1. Lie down to go to sleep only when sleepy.
2. Do not use the bed for anything except sleeping.
3. If you go to bed and cannot fall asleep within about 10 minutes, get up, go to another room, and stay up until you feel sleepy.
4. If you still cannot fall asleep, repeat step 3 as often as necessary.
5. Set your alarm and get up at the same time every morning, regardless of the amount of sleep you have had.
6. Do not nap during the day.

Sleep medications should be used rarely and only on a temporary basis because of their diminishing effectiveness over time and potential harmful effect. The use of alcohol and caffeine after noon should be strongly discouraged.

EXCESSIVE SLEEPINESS

Narrowing down and diagnosis

Narrowing down the problem of excessive sleepiness consists of distinguishing among problems that are due to not enough sleep, normal variation in sleep patterns, depression, drug use, apnea, narcolepsy, and physical illness (Table 18-2).

Excessive sleepiness due to lack of sleep should be the first hypothesis. A careful history of the problem, focussing on hours of sleep, is important. Since there is no right amount of sleep, a trial of increasing sleep time is the best diagnostic method if sleep deprivation is suspected. Chronic sleep deprivation has been suggested to be a fact of modern life for many adolescents and adults (3,19). As well, it appears that daytime sleepiness may be a normal response to the onset of puberty (20).

Excessive sleepiness due to depression should be accompanied by other signs of depression. Excessive sleepiness due to drug use disrupting sleep or inducing daytime sleepiness is best determined by direct questioning. Requests for long-term prescription of mood-modifying drugs also warn of inappropriate drug use.

Narcolepsy usually presents as excessive daytime sleepiness and sudden muscle weakness following an unexpected stimulus or emotion, such as laughter or fear (cataplexy) (3). Narcolepsy is a genetic disorder of rapid eye movement sleep that peaks in onset at between 15 and 25 years of age. The syndrome is characterized by irresistible sleepiness that develops 3 to 4 hours

Table 18-2. Problems of excessive sleepiness

Type	Age	Narrowing down	Management
Sleep-deprived	All ages	No other symptoms; late nights; responds to more sleep	More sleep
Normal	All ages	No illnesses or other symptoms; frequent at puberty	Reassurance
Depression	6 years and up	Other symptoms of depression	Treat depression
Drug-induced	All ages	Direct questioning re drug or alcohol use	Reduce drug or alcohol use
Apnea	All ages	Loud snoring; stopping breathing during sleep for more than 15–20 seconds; learning problems	Referral to consultant
Narcolepsy	15 years and up	Sleep attacks; cataplexy; hypnagogic hallucinations	Referral to consultant

after waking, hypnagogic hallucinations (single images that occur when falling asleep), cataplexy, and disrupted night sleep.

Narcolepsy is frequently misdiagnosed as schizophrenia (because of the hypnagogic hallucinations), or learning disability (5 to 15 second microsleeps interfere with learning), or plain laziness. Close questioning of the parents about similar problems in other family members and careful discussions with the child can help narrow down the problem, but diagnosis will require somnographic recording by a consultant.

Excessive sleepiness due to the apnea-hypersomnia syndrome is evidenced by excessive sleepiness and poor nighttime sleep. Declines in school performance, abnormal daytime behavior, secondary enuresis, morning headache, and progressive development of hypertension combined with *loud* snoring constitute the clinical symtomatology (21). As mentioned earlier, this condition is rare in childhood. Apnea can be timed by the parents; period of sleep apnea of less than 15 to 20 seconds are normal. If the apnea is longer than 15 seconds, the child should be referred to a consultant, who may order somnographic recording.

Excessive sleepiness due to illness should be accompanied by other symptoms or signs of underlying illness.

Management of excessive sleepiness

The management of excessive sleepiness depends on the cause of the problem. Excessive sleepiness due to lack of sleep is best managed by more sleep, but compliance with this recommendation may be problematic.

Excessive sleepiness due to depression is best treated by psychological or pharmacologic treatment of the depression (see Chapter 23). Narcolepsy-induced sleepiness is usually managed by a consultant who may use stimulant medication, often in conjunction with a tricyclic antidepressant (NO CLEAR EVIDENCE).

Apnea-hypersomnia is usually managed by a consultant. Surgical treatment by adenoidectomy and tonsillectomy (21) has been used in obstructive apnea. Careful documentation that apnea is indeed occurring is essential before surgery is considered. Central apnea may be medically managed with tricyclic antidepressants or stimulants (NO CLEAR EVIDENCE).

PROBLEMS WITH THE SLEEP-WAKE SCHEDULE

Narrowing down and diagnosis

Many parents complain that their infant or toddler is not on the same sleep-wake schedule that they are, that is, the child sleeps during the day and stays awake during the night. Parents may also complain about the same behavior in their teenaged children. The problem may be manifested as difficulty in falling asleep without subsequent difficulty in maintaining sleep. Narrowing down the problem is seldom difficult, and the behavior is a problem only when the child is disruptive, is endangered during nighttime forays, or does not fulfill expected obligations because of tiredness or sleeping late.

Management of problems with the sleep-wake schedule

Management of problems with the sleep-wake schedule in children should focus on establishing clear cues for bedtime by providing a consistent, quiet, bedtime routine. Napping should be eliminated. Management should also ensure the safety of the child; in cases in which the child's wandering at night is dangerous, it may be necessary to install latches or warning buzzers on the child's bedroom door.

There is SUGGESTIVE EVIDENCE that the delayed sleep phase syndrome can be treated in adults by "chronotherapy" in which the internal clock is reset by delaying sleep for 3 hours each "day" until the appropriate bedtime is reached. After this, a rigid routine is followed (22).

EPISODIC EVENTS DURING SLEEP (PARASOMNIAS)

Narrowing down and diagnosis

Episodic events during sleep (parasomnias) include: bed-wetting (see Chapter 10), sleepwalking, sleep-talking, head-banging, and teeth-grinding. Narrowing down the problem involves distinguishing the different parasomnias from each other and from more serious disorders, such as nocturnal epilepsy.

Sleepwalking and sleep-talking occur at all ages, may run in families, and are not due to organic or psychological conditions. They may be triggered in predisposed individuals by stress. Usually, sleepwalking and sleep-talking are readily distinguished from epilepsy and dissociative states, without resorting to an electroencephalogram; doubtful cases can be referred to a consultant.

Sleep-talking consists of short, incomprehensible statements or jumbled words. Dissociative states are rare and are marked by longer, more psychologically meaningful talking that is frequently goal-oriented. Dissociative states are accompanied by other evidence of serious psychological disturbance. Nocturnal epilepsy is often accompanied by an interictal electroencephalogram with epileptiform discharges, a strong family history of epilepsy, seizurelike behavior during the attacks, and epileptic seizures during the day. However, only the electroencephalographic recording of a frank epileptic discharge is firmly diagnostic (23).

Reports of "bad dreams" may be due to hypnagogic hallucinations, nightmares, or night terrors. Careful questioning will determine the nature and time of the "bad dream" (Table 18-3). Hypnagogic hallucinations occur on

Table 18-3. Problems with bad dreams

Type	Age	Narrowing down	Management
Nightmares	All ages	Well-formed content	Treat anxiety
Night terrors	All ages	Very high arousal, no clear content, no real wakening, not consolable	Reassurance of parents; diazepam or triazolam at bedtime if terrors occur more than three times a week
Hypnagogic hallucinations	All ages	Occur at falling asleep or waking; may be accompanied by cataplexy	Reassurance if infrequent; suspect narcolepsy if frequent

falling asleep or on waking, are often accompanied by cataplexy, consist of a single image, and, if infrequent, are normal. They are frightening experiences and children may fight sleep to avoid them. Hypnagogic hallucinations that occur frequently (several times per week) are suggestive of narcolepsy.

Nightmares occur during rapid eye movement sleep (at least 30 to 45 minutes after the initiation of sleep) and the images are well formulated and often follow a story line. Children waking from nightmares are often upset but are consolable. Children may develop fear of going to bed after intense nightmares. Occasional nightmares are normal; nightmares that occur more than once a week may be the result of specific feelings of anxiety, insecurity, or stress.

Night terrors occur after a period of sleep, usually in the first third of the night, and bring the child to a very high state of arousal. Screaming, a racing heart rate, sweating, and pallor are frequent accompaniments. The child is usually inconsolable, does not appear to be fully awake, and returns to sleep after the terror. Only rarely will the child have any memory of the event in the morning. Childhood-onset night terrors are not usually indicative of psychopathology but may emerge under stress in predisposed individuals.

Head-banging or rocking prior to sleep onset are habitual, comforting strategies that usually disappear in deep sleep. Retarded or disturbed children may continue the rocking or head-banging throughout deeper sleep. Teeth-grinding during sleep is not indicative of any psychological problem and is readily diagnosed on the basis of the parents' report.

Management of episodic events during sleep

The management of sleepwalking should focus on safety. Children who are sleepwalking can seriously harm themselves by walking into the street or falling down stairs. Locks on doors and windows and a warning buzzer for the parents may be required. Diazepam (1 to 20 milligrams at bedtime) (15) or triazolam (0.25 milligrams), which is eliminated more rapidly (24), may be helpful in severe, intractable cases (SUGGESTIVE EVIDENCE). There is no management available or required for sleep-talking.

The management of nightmares, if they are infrequent, consists of reassuring the parents and comforting the child. In some cases in which triggering events, such as parental arguments or scary television shows, can be identified, removal of the trigger is the obvious strategy. Children with frequent, severe nightmares often need a consultant's help in dealing with anxiety.

Night terrors require ample reassurance of the parents. The blood-curdling scream of a child can terrify even the most confident parent. Safety of the child should be ensured, since sleepwalking may occur at the same time. In severe cases, diazepam (1 to 20 milligrams at bedtime) (15) or triazolam (0.25 milligrams) (24) can be prescribed (SUGGESTIVE EVIDENCE).

Head-banging or rocking at sleep onset is best ignored. Padding of the bed or bolting of the bed to the floor may be required for safety. A firm "Stop that!" may help (NO CLEAR EVIDENCE).

Teeth-grinding during the night in children usually requires no intervention unless there is damage to the teeth or pain. A consultant's treatment may be dental splinting or correction of bite, or psychological stress management (NO CLEAR EVIDENCE).

REFERENCES

1. Diagnostic classification of sleep and arousal disorders of the Association of Sleep Disorders Centers and the Association for the Psychophysiological Study of Sleep. *Sleep* 2:1–137, 1979.
2. Anders, T.A. Night waking in infants during the first year of life. *Pediatrics* 63:860–864, 1979.
3. Anders, T.F., Carskadon, M.A., Dement, W.C. Sleep and sleepiness in children and adolescents. *Pediatr. Clin. North Am.* 27:29–43, 1980.
4. Moore, T., Ucko, L.E. Night waking in early infancy: Part 1. *Arch. Dis. Child.* 32:333–342, 1957.
5. Salzarulo, P., Chevalier, A. Sleep problems in children and their relationship with early disturbances of the waking-sleeping rhythms. *Sleep* 6:47–51, 1983.
6. Price, V.A., Coates, T.J., Thoresen C.E., Grinstead, O.A. Prevalence and correlates of poor sleep among adolescents. *Am. J. Dis. Child.* 132:583–586, 1978.
7. Carey, W.B. Night waking and temperament in infancy. *J. Pediatr.* 84:756–758, 1974.
8. Osterholm, P., Lindeke, L.L., Amidon, D. Sleep disturbance in infants aged 6 to 12 months. *Pediatric Nursing* 269–271, 1983.
9. Blurton-Jones, N., Rosetti-Ferreira, M.C., Farquar-Brown, M., Macdonald, L. The association between perinatal factors and later night waking. *Dev. Med. Child Neurol.* 20:427–434, 1978.

10. Guilleminault, C., Anders, T.F. Sleep disorders in children. *Adv. Pediatr.* 22:151–174, 1976.
11. Weissbluth, M. *Crybabies: Coping with Colic.* New York, Arbor House, 1984.
12. Christophersen, E.R. Incorporating behavioral pediatrics into primary care. *Pediatr. Clin. North Am.* 29:261–296, 1982.
13. Jones, D.P.H., Verduyn, C.M. Behavioural management of sleep problems. *Arch. Dis. Child.* 58:442–444, 1983.
14. Richman, N., Douglas, J., Hunt, H., Lansdown, R., Levere, R. Behavioral methods in the treatment of sleep disorders—A pilot study. *J. Child Psychol. Psychiatry* 26:581–590, 1985.
15. White, J.H. Psychopharmacology in childhood: Current status and future prospectives. *Psychiatr. Clin. North Am.* 3:443–453, 1980.
16. Russo, R.M., Gururaj, V.J., Allen, J.E. The effectiveness of diphenhydramine HCl in pediatric sleep disorders. *J. Clin. Pharmacol.* 16:284–288, 1976.
17. Richman, N. A double blind drug trial of sleep problems in young children. *J. Child Psychol. Psychiatry* 26:591–598, 1985.
18. Bootzin, R.R., Nicassio, P.M. Behavioral treatments for insomnia. In *Progress in Behavior Modification*, vol. 6, Hersen, M., Eisler, R.M., Miller, P., eds. New York: Academic Press, 1978, pp. 1–45.
19. Webb, W., Agnew, H. Are we chronically sleep deprived? *Bulletin of the Psychonomic Society* 6:47–48, 1975.
20. Pivik, R.T. Order and disorder during sleep ontogeny: A selective review. In *Advances in Behavioral Medicine for Children and Adolescents*, Firestone, P., McGrath, P.J., Feldman, W., eds. Hillsdale, N.J.: Lawrence Erlbaum Associates, 1983, pp. 75–102.
21. Guilleminault, C., Eldridge, F.L., Simmons, F.B., Dement, W.C. Sleep apnea in eight children. *Pediatrics* 58:23–30, 1976.
22. Czeisler, C., Richardson, G., Coleman, R., Zimmerman, J., Moore-Ede, M., Dement, W., Weitzman, E. Chronotherapy; Resetting the circadian clocks of patients with delayed sleep phase insomnia. *Sleep* 4:1–21, 1981.
23. Gastaut, H., Broughton, R. *Epileptic Seizures: Clinical and Electrographic Features, Diagnosis and Treatment.* Springfield, Ill.: Charles Thomas, 1972.
24. Greenblatt, D.J., Shader, R.S., Abernethy, D.R. Drug therapy: Current status of benzodiazepines. *N. Engl. J. Med.* 309:355–358, 1983.

19

SHORTNESS AND THINNESS

Children can be too short, too fat, too thin, or too tall. What does "too" mean? It can mean too short statistically, based on age-related norms; too short for the familial pattern of height but within the age-related norms; or too short for individual, familial, or societal preferences. In assessing a child with a growth problem, the physician must evaluate the child's height and weight in relation to those of other children of the same age and in relation to those of the rest of the family; in addition, he or she must determine whether the problem is due to illness, or nutritional deficiency or excess, or, if not, is of sufficient magnitude to produce stress in the child and/or the family.

PREVALENCE

Using strict statistical definitions, problems of height or weight are limited to those that fall outside two standard deviations from the mean. This is obviously inappropriate, since by this definition any 16-year-old boy more than 6 foot, 1 inch tall would be considered "abnormal." On the contrary, it is desirable, in our culture, for a male teenager to be tall. A 16-year-old girl, on the other hand, who is close to 6 feet in height would be "abnormal" in the statistical sense and consider herself a freak because she is so much taller than most girls her age, yet she could be perfectly healthy.

For practical purposes, therefore, this discussion deals mainly with the major reasons that children with growth problems are taken to physicians, that is, children who are too thin or too short. Obesity is discussed in Chapter 17. The age groups considered are infancy, preschool-aged, school-aged, and adolescence. Narrowing down, diagnosis, and management are inextricably linked with regard to shortness and thinness, since diagnosis of the major causes of both is often made after the results of an intervention are observed. For example, a benign cause of shortness can be diagnosed if the management decision was merely to assess the growth velocity in 6 months and normal growth occurred.

163

TOO THIN

Infancy

The most common growth problem in this age group occurs in the infant who is too thin for his or her height. The typical growth curve shows the child to be at or above the tenth percentile for height but below the third percentile in weight. This is generally called failure to thrive.

Failure to thrive in infants is due to either inadequate nutrition or adequate intake of nutrients but inadequate absorption (Table 19–1). Clues in the history and physical examination are helpful in narrowing down the problem. Poverty is relatively easy to assess. Parental depression or poor parenting may be more difficult. If the child's general developmental level is normal, neglect or deprivation is unlikely. The parents may be attentive and loving but not able to provide adequate nutrition, or the child's problem may be malabsorption. A history of chronic diarrhea and a falling-off in weight after the introduction of wheat into the diet suggests celiac disease. A history of chronic cough or one or more bouts of pneumonia may indicate cystic fibrosis.

In one study, in 82% of 185 children admitted to a children's hospital with failure to thrive there was no organic etiology. In all 18% of children in whom

Table 19-1. Diagnosis and management of failure to thrive

	Possible causes	Clinical clues	Intervention
Inadequate intake of nutrients	Poverty	Appearance of infant, social history	Social service assessment; follow-up to monitor physical and mental growth
	Maternal depression	Postpartum mood change in mother	Social and psychiatric assessment; careful follow-up
	Poor parenting skills	Unwed or immature parent, no support to parent; history of deprivation as a child	Social service assessment; careful follow-up to monitor parent-child relationship and growth and development
	Chewing or swallowing problems	Cerebral palsy; cleft palate	Referral to cerebral palsy center; dental prosthesis, surgery
Inadequate absorption of nutrients	Celiac disease	Weight gain poor after solid foods started, chronic diarrhea	Referral for studies, jejunal biopsy
	Cystic fibrosis	Chronic chest problem	Sweat test, chest films; referral to cystic fibrosis clinic

there was a clear-cut physical cause, the diagnosis was suspected on the basis of the history and physical examination. Although each infant underwent a mean of more than ten laboratory tests, fewer than 2% of the tests were of diagnostic value, and then only when indicated by a specific clue from the history and physical examination (1). Although the list of organic causes of failure to gain weight is very long, the family physician is not likely to see many of the uncommon conditions and is unlikely to miss them during a careful clinical assessment.

If there is environment deprivation, an infant's development may be delayed. Such children often smile less, are apathetic, and display a form of unusual watchfulness that has been described as "radar-like" (2). Parents are often frightened to give an accurate history of the child's poor diet and lack of environmental stimulation. Management almost always includes hospitalization of 1 or more weeks for both diagnostic and therapeutic purposes. Laboratory investigations need be considered only if adequate nutrition, assessed daily by a nutritionist, is not associated with weight gain within 1 to 2 weeks. Often the infant will become more alert and show catch-up growth not only physically but also mentally. This is especially so if nurses and child-life workers engage the infant in age-appropriate play and provide warmth and cuddling.

A consultation with a social worker is indicated if environmental deprivation is suspected. If, during a short hospitalization, the child shows physical and mental growth, then the diagnosis of deprivation is secure. Consultants in social service, and possibly psychology and psychiatry, will be helpful when the child is discharged from the hospital. The physician's role then is to ensure that appropriate physical and mental growth proceed and that the parents comply with the consultants' recommendations.

Preschool-aged

The same physical causes that lead to thinness in infants may produce thinness in preschool-aged children. Failure to thrive because of psychosocial reasons does not often begin after infancy. The declining appetite of 2-year-olds often worries parents; this is physiological and is associated with the normal slowing of the growth rate after the first year of life. Occasionally, this parental anxiety can result in a power struggle over eating, which can cause the toddler to eat so little that his or her weight gain is poor. This problem is discussed more completely in Chapter 17. Rarely, chronic diseases of the kidneys, heart, or lungs may cause inadequate weight gain, but there are almost always clinical clues pointing to these (see Chapters 7, 9, and 10).

School-aged

In addition to the medical conditions already described, malabsorption due to chronic inflammatory bowel disease (Crohn's disease, ulcerative colitis) and hyperthyroidism may cause poor weight gain or weight loss in school-aged children. Those with inflammatory bowel disease almost always have abdominal pain, blood in the stools, diarrhea, or sufficient weakness and lethargy in addition to their weight problem that the physician should be highly suspicious. Referral to a pediatric consultant who treats children with these conditions is indicated.

Children who are hyperthyroid burn their calories inefficiently; thus, although their intake may be more than adequate and their absorption normal, they do not gain weight and may lose weight. Symptoms of anxiety, palpitations, staring or bulging eyes, rapid pulse, heat intolerance, enlarged thyroid gland, restlessness, poor concentration, and weakness should lead to the diagnosis. Serum thyroxine levels will be abnormal and this finding should prompt referral to a consultant.

Adolescence

In addition to the above-mentioned medical conditions, anorexia nervosa is becoming a relatively common problem causing excessive weight loss in teenagers (see Chapter 17).

TOO SHORT

Infancy

It is unusual to see infants who are too short for their age and weight. Aside from familial short stature and familial slow maturation, medical causes of shortness in infancy are rare (Table 19-2).

Preschool-aged

It is not common for preschool-aged children to have a problem of short stature, since many physicians do not regularly measure height in this age group and many parents do not have the opportunity to compare the stature of their toddlers with that of other toddlers (see Table 19-2).

School-aged

Once short children enter school, they and their parents often become concerned that they are not as tall as their peers. Table 19-2 can be used as a guide for handling shortness in children in all age groups.

Adolescence

Adolescent males who are "too short" are usually short because their parents are (familial short stature) or because puberty and the pubertal growth spurt are delayed (familial slow maturation). Most other causes listed in Table 19-2 will have been sorted out by the time of adolescence.

Table 19-2. Diagnosis and management of short stature

Possible causes	Clinical clues	Intervention
Familial short stature	Normal activity and appetite; healthy; family history of shortness	Reassurance; monitor growth velocity; referral if growth in next 6 months is 2 cm or less (at age 4 or more)
Familial slow maturation	Family history of delayed puberty and delayed growth spurt, but normal ultimate height	Reassuance; monitor growth velocity; rarely, give androgens to boys; referral if growth in next 6 months is 2 cm or less (at age 4 or more)
Hormone problem Too little growth hormone	Normal family history; very slow rate of growth; tend to be chubby and very far below third percentile in height; normal body proportions	Radiographs for bone age; referral to consultant for growth hormone assay
Too little thyroid hormone	Low activity level, slow pulse, cold intolerance, constipation	Measure serum T_4 T S H, and thyroid antibody levels; referral to consultant
Too much cortisone	Cushing's syndrome; history of taking steroids	Referral to consultant
Chromosomal problems (girls)	Web neck, shield chest, increased carrying angle of arms, absence of sexual development, extreme short stature, otherwise well-nourished; or, extreme short stature in a well-nourished girl	Blood test for chromosome analysis; referral to pediatric or gynecologic consultant experienced in dealing with Turner's syndrome
Skeletal problem, e.g., achondroplasia	Disproportionate shortness of limbs	Radiographs; genetic and psychosocial counseling; self-help group (Little People of America)
Chronic medical condition	Symptoms or signs referable to heart, lungs, genitourinary, or gastrointestinal system	Confirmation by laboratory; referral to consultant

T_4, thyroxine; TSH, thyroid-stimulating hormone.

As is clear from Table 19-2, we do not suggest bone-age radiographs when familial short stature or familial slow maturation is suspected. One major pediatric textbook does recommend radiographic assessment of skeletal age in adolescents (3). If the history is suggestive and the activity level and appetite appropriate, and the physical examination reveals a perfectly healthy child or adolescent, a repeat, accurate height measurement in 6 months that demonstrates normal growth velocity provides much more information than can any laboratory test.

Normal growth velocity means that the child is absorbing an adequate amount of nutrients and has normal endocrine function. If the height is substantially below the third percentile and there is little evidence of growth in the preceding year or two, as manifested by little change in clothes or shoe size, a radiograph for bone age is indicated at the first visit. Tanner and Whitehouse (4) published valuable charts of weight and height growth velocity for boys and girls. As a general rule of thumb, a child more than 5 years old who is growing at least 2 to 3 centimeters every six months does not need to undergo any laboratory investigation. In adolescents, evidence of sexual maturation commensurate with age (5) is reassurance that a growth spurt is likely. If sexual maturation is not starting by age 14, referral to a consultant is indicated.

In the future, boys with familial short stature may be considered for treatment with synthetic human growth hormone, should it become readily available and affordable, but for the moment, they and their parents can only be reassured that they are healthy, normal (in a health sense if not in a statistical sense), and will be able to do everything that their taller counterparts can (with the possible exception of becoming professional basketball players). The physician should be available to listen to their descriptions of disappointment and understand how much physical appearance means to teenagers (and their parents) in our society.

Teenage boys with familial slow maturation will often be reassured when it is pointed out to them that their fathers or uncles also did not have a growth spurt or develop facial hair or big muscles until they were 15 or 16 years old. Some 15- or 16-year-old boys begin to show signs of anxiety and/or depression because of their presumed lack of virility; for them, a consultation for consideration of exogenous androgen therapy to speed up the onset and progress of puberty may be considered.

Short teenage girls (unless they are very short) rarely complain to a physician about this as a problem, because short stature in girls and women in our culture is not as great a cosmetic handicap.

REFERENCES

1. Sills, R.H. Failure to thrive. The role of clinical and laboratory evaluation. *Am. J. Dis. Child.* 132:967–969, 1978.
2. Goldbloom, R.B. Failure to thrive. *Pediatr. Clin. North Am.* 29:151–166, 1982.
3. Behrman, R.E., Baughan, V.C., III, eds., *Nelson's Textbook of Pediatrics*, 12th ed. Philadelphia: W.B. Saunders, 1983, p. 43.
4. Tanner, J.M., Whitehouse, R.H. Longitudinal standards for height, weight, height velocity, weight velocity and stages of puberty. *Arch. Dis. Child.* 51:170, 1976.
5. Smith, D.W. *Growth and Its Disorders.* Philadelphia: W.B. Saunders, 1977, pp. 70–76.

20

BEHAVIOR PROBLEMS

Problems with behavior can be divided into two categories: oversocialization or internalizing disorders, in which anxiety and depression play a major role, and undersocialization or externalizing disorders, which are characterized by noncompliance with adults' requests. Internalizing problems are discussed in Chapter 23. This chapter focuses on externalizing disorders, which include behavior problems, particularly noncompliance in otherwise normal children; conduct disorders; Attention Deficit Disorder (with or without hyperactivity); difficult temperament; and problems caused by parents' setting unrealistic standards for their child's behavior. Behavior problems associated with sleep are discussed in Chapter 18, and behavior problems at mealtimes are reviewed in Chapter 17.

PREVALENCE

Virtually all children display some difficult behaviors at some time. Indeed, total compliance with parental requests is not an accepted norm in our society (1,2). Noncompliance is the most common problem cited by parents who seek help at pediatric clinics and treatment programs (3). There are no data on how many parents seek help for their normal children's occasional behavior problems.

The prevalence of conduct disorders has been estimated to be between 1.7% for 10-year-old girls living in a semirural setting to about 12% for inner-city, 10-year-old boys (4–6).

The prevalence of Attention Deficit Disorder has been estimated to be between 2 and 20%, depending on the criteria used. Most investigators suggest that 3 to 5% of school-aged children have this disorder, with a 6:1 predominance in boys (7). Attention Deficit Disorder (8) is the current diagnostic term for what used to be called hyperactivity. The term is more accurate because lack of attention is the primary element of the disorder. Children can have Attention Deficit Disorder with or without excessive motor activity (hyperactivity).

Temperament refers to the characteristic style of response that a child displays in a wide variety of situations. Temperament is biological in origin and, although it can be somewhat modified by experience, is enduring. Three major constellations of temperament have been identified. "Easy" children (approximately 40% of children) develop regular sleeping and feeding schedules quickly, take to new foods easily, smile at strangers, and accept new situations easily. "Difficult" children (approximately 10% of children) have irregular feeding and sleeping schedules, are slow to accept new routines, people, and situations, cry frequently, and often have temper tantrums. "Slow to warm up" children (approximately 15% of children) have mild negative responses to new situations and some biological irregularity (9).

The prevalence of parents' having unrealistic expectations for their child's behavior is not known. The overlap among these categories of problems is considerable (10).

NARROWING DOWN AND DIAGNOSIS OF BEHAVIOR PROBLEMS

In primary care, the only method of narrowing down behavior problems is to obtain information from parents, baby-sitters, the child, and teachers or day-care staff. It is crucial to remember that the behavior a child displays in the consulting room often does not reflect his or her behavior elsewhere. Standardized behavior checklists such as the Eyberg Child Behavior Inventory (11,12) are particularly helpful. The Eyberg inventory is shown in Table 20–1, which can be photo-copied for use in the office.

Because a mother and father often have very different views of their child's behavior, it is wise to have both parents independently complete the inventory. Scanning the two inventories can quickly reveal what behaviors are seen by each of the parents to be difficult.

Following an initial consultation about the behavior problem, it is useful to have parents complete a week-long log of the antecedents and consequences of the behavior problem, as in the example below:

Name _____

DATE	What happened before problem?	Problem	What happened then?	Eventual outcome
Jan. 2	I asked Tim to pick up toys.	Tim ignored my request.	Asked again, about 10 times.	He picked up toys. I was very angry.

Completion of the behavior log frequently helps parents change their approach to a problem by allowing them to reflect on patterns that become evi-

Table 20-1. Eyberg child behavior inventory

Directions: Below are a series of phrases that describe children's behavior. Please (**1**) circle the number describing **how often** the behavior **currently** occurs with your child, and (**2**) circle either "yes" **or** "no" to indicate whether the behavior is **currently a problem.**

	How often does this occur with your child?							Is this a problem for you?	
	Never	*Seldom*	*Sometimes*		*Often*		*Always*		
1. Dawdles in getting dressed	1	2	3	4	5	6	7	Yes	No
2. Dawdles or lingers at mealtime	1	2	3	4	5	6	7	Yes	No
3. Has poor table manners	1	2	3	4	5	6	7	Yes	No
4. Refuses to eat food presented	1	2	3	4	5	6	7	Yes	No
5. Refuses to do chores when asked	1	2	3	4	5	6	7	Yes	No
6. Slow in getting ready for bed	1	2	3	4	5	6	7	Yes	No
7. Refuses to go to bed on time	1	2	3	4	5	6	7	Yes	No
8. Does not obey house rules on his own	1	2	3	4	5	6	7	Yes	No
9. Refuses to obey until threatened with punishment	1	2	3	4	5	6	7	Yes	No
10. Acts defiant when told to do something	1	2	3	4	5	6	7	Yes	No
11. Argues with parents about rules	1	2	3	4	5	6	7	Yes	No
12. Gets angry when doesn't get his own way	1	2	3	4	5	6	7	Yes	No
13. Has temper tantrums	1	2	3	4	5	6	7	Yes	No
14. Sasses adults	1	2	3	4	5	6	7	Yes	No
15. Whines	1	2	3	4	5	6	7	Yes	No
16. Cries easily	1	2	3	4	5	6	7	Yes	No
17. Yells or screams	1	2	3	4	5	6	7	Yes	No
18. Hits parents	1	2	3	4	5	6	7	Yes	No
19. Destroys toys and other objects	1	2	3	4	5	6	7	Yes	No
20. Is careless with toys and other objects	1	2	3	4	5	6	7	Yes	No
21. Steals	1	2	3	4	5	6	7	Yes	No
22. Lies	1	2	3	4	5	6	7	Yes	No
23. Teases or provokes other children	1	2	3	4	5	6	7	Yes	No
24. Verbally fights with friends his own age	1	2	3	4	5	6	7	Yes	No
25. Verbally fights with sisters and brothers	1	2	3	4	5	6	7	Yes	No

Table 20-1. Eyberg child behavior inventory   (cont'd.)

26. Physically fights with friends his own age	1	2	3	4	5	6	7		Yes	No
27. Physically fights with sisters and brothers	1	2	3	4	5	6	7		Yes	No
28. Constantly seeks attention	1	2	3	4	5	6	7		Yes	No
29. Interrupts	1	2	3	4	5	6	7		Yes	No
30. Is easily distracted	1	2	3	4	5	6	7		Yes	No
31. Has short attention span	1	2	3	4	5	6	7		Yes	No
32. Fails to finish tasks or projects	1	2	3	4	5	6	7		Yes	No
33. Has difficulty entertaining himself alone	1	2	3	4	5	6	7		Yes	No
34. Has difficulty concentrating on one thing	1	2	3	4	5	6	7		Yes	No
35. Is overactive or restless	1	2	3	4	5	6	7		Yes	No
36. Wets the bed	1	2	3	4	5	6	7		Yes	No

Reprinted with permission of Sheila Eyberg, Ph.D., and *J. Clin. Child Psychol.*

dent. As well, the logs can become the focus of discussion about what can be done differently either to avoid future incidents or to handle them when they arise (NO CLEAR EVIDENCE).

Behavior problems in normal children

There are no universally agreed-upon criteria for how much a normal child should comply with parental requests. Family values and the specific areas of noncompliance both influence the rate of noncompliance tolerated. Research on "normal" families suggests that the level of normal noncompliance is approximately 8% (13). Frequently, it becomes quite clear that the problem is that of a poor parent-child match. For example, a normal but active 5-year-old might be no problem for a tolerant but firm parent, but could well be the nemesis of an anxious, unassertive parent. Similarly, parental, especially maternal, depression or marital discord may make "normal misbehavior" virtually impossible for a parent to handle (3). Some theorists see any child misbehavior as evidence of family dysfunction that should be treated with family therapy. We see the issue more simply as a lack of appropriate parental skills for dealing with the child's behavior, until there is some clear indication to the contrary (NO CLEAR EVIDENCE).

Conduct disorders

The main symptom of a conduct disorder is a repetitive and persistent pattern of violation of the basic rights of society or other individuals (8). Examples of this type of behavior include repetitive stealing, both within the home and outside the home; chronic lying; the repeated setting of fires; and frequent aggression. Diagnosis is usually made by a consultant.

Attention Deficit Disorder (hyperactivity)

The essential diagnostic criteria for Attention Deficit Disorder are impulsivity and inattention. Table 20–2 details the criteria for Attention Deficit Disorder given in the *Diagnostic and Statistical Manual of Mental Disorders* (third edition). The overlap between Attention Deficit Disorder and conduct disorder has been reported to be between 30 and 65% (10).

Difficult temperament

The diagnosis of difficult temperament can be made using the temperament scales devised by Carey (14) or on the basis of a careful history of the child's behavior. Difficulties with behavior in children less than 18 months old should not be seen as a behavior problem but a manifestation of *normal* variations in temperament.

Table 20-2. Diagnostic criteria for Attention Deficit Disorder (appropriate for children over 5 years of age)

Inattention—at least three of the following:
1. Often fails to finish things he or she starts.
2. Often doesn't seem to listen.
3. Is easily distracted.
4. Has difficulty concentrating on schoolwork or other tasks that require sustained attention.
5. Has difficulty sticking to a play activity.

Impulsivity—at least three of the following:
1. Often acts before thinking.
2. Shifts excessively from one activity to another.
3. Has difficulty organizing work (this not being due to cognitive impairment).
4. Needs a lot of supervision.
5. Frequently calls out in class.
6. Has difficulty awaiting turn in games or group situations.

Hyperactivity—at least two of the following:
1. Runs about or climbs on things excessively.
2. Has difficulty sitting still or fidgets excessively
3. Has difficulty staying seated.
4. Moves about excessively during sleep.
5. Is always "on the go" or acts as if "driven by a motor."

Reprinted with permission.

Unrealistic parental expectations

Determining that parents have unrealistic expectations of their child's behavior is difficult, but it can be done by reviewing some of the incidents of "misbehavior" recounted by the parent or recorded in the behavior log. In addition, one can ask specific questions geared to the age of the child, such as, "Do you think there is anything wrong with punishing a 9-month-old for crying?" or "Do you think a 3-year-old can be expected to play quietly for an hour or so when his or her mother is not feeling well?" or "Should a 5-year-old be expected to help by feeding, dressing, and changing diapers for an infant?" (15).

The assertions of parents with children less than 18 months old who describe their child's behavior as deliberate disobedience aimed at getting the parents angry should be taken very seriously. Labeling this type of behavior as disobedience in children this young is most inappropriate, and such parents may be at higher risk of abusing their children (15).

MANAGEMENT OF BEHAVIOR PROBLEMS

Behavior problems in normal children

Families who have difficulties managing the behavior of their normal children can benefit from the assistance of their physician. Treatment of mild behavior problems is well within the scope and capabilities of primary care physicians, whereas treatment of more severe behavior problems is probably not. Severe problems are best treated by consultants (16). The determination of what constitutes a "more severe" behavior problem is difficult and depends on the interest and skill of the primary care physician, the availability of alternative treatment, and the family's response to initial attempts to help.

There is FIRM EVIDENCE supporting the effectiveness of a treatment program for noncompliant behavior (3) consisting of teaching a variety of skills to the parents through discussion, role playing, and rehearsal. The skills are taught in the following order:

1. Pay attention to the child's neutral or positive behavior.
2. Ignore minor misbehavior.
3. Use continuous reinforcement to establish appropriate behavior.
4. Use intermittent reinforcement to maintain appropriate behavior.
5. Give clear, specific commands.
6. Use "time out" for noncompliance.

This treatment has been delivered by specially trained therapists in ten 1-hour sessions. Although there is NO CLEAR EVIDENCE of the effectiveness of the program when delivered by primary care physicians in fewer or shorter sessions, it may be worthwhile for the physician to use these principles in advising parents.

Christophersen (16,17) devised handouts for physicians to use when advising parents about specific behavior problems. There is SUGGESTIVE EVIDENCE that these may be effective.

Marital therapy or treatment or maternal depression when indicated may alter the behavior problems of the child (NO CLEAR EVIDENCE).

Conduct disorders

Long-term intensive behavior therapy for families in a sophisticated research setting (18,19) has been shown to be effective (FIRM EVIDENCE) in the treatment of conduct disorders. However, treatment by primary care physicians has not been investigated, and children with such problems should be referred as early as possible to a consultant for intensive management.

The primary care physician can play a major role in identifying the problem and in obtaining appropriate referral for children with conduct disorders and in providing encouragement to the family coping with these very difficult problems.

There is SUGGESTIVE EVIDENCE (18) of the effectiveness of stimulant medication (methylphenidate and pemoline) in children with conduct disorders.

"Toughlove" (20) is a self-help program for parents of children with conduct disorders. The emphasis is on support by other parents and firm consequences for noncompliance in teenagers with conduct disorders. At this time, there is NO CLEAR EVIDENCE of its effectiveness. Similarly, there is NO CLEAR EVIDENCE that psychotherapy or in-patient residential treatment is effective.

Attention Deficit Disorder

Attention Deficit Disorder can be managed either pharmacologically or psychologically or by a combination of the two. Methylphenidate is the drug of choice, but pemoline and D-amphetamine have also been used. Doses of methylphenidate should be 0.3 to 1 mg/kg, beginning with the lower dose and titrating upward until there is positive response or negative side effects. The dose range for D-amphetamine is 0.15 to 0.5 mg/kg, and for pemoline, 0.5 to 2 mg/kg (7). A child who does not respond or who experiences severe side effects on one drug may do well on one of the others. Imipramine has also been recommended for children with attention deficit disorder (7). Pharmacological therapy is not recommended for preschool-aged children.

There is FIRM EVIDENCE (21,22) of the efficacy of stimulant medication for the short-term alleviation (i.e., several months) of the behavior problems of school-aged children with Attention Deficit Disorder. There is SUGGES-TIVE EVIDENCE (23) that stimulant medication may have similar positive effects for short-term academic deficiencies. However, there is NO CLEAR EVIDENCE of long-term effectiveness of stimulant medication or the use of stimulants in preschool-aged children (7). A major problem with stimulant medication, as with all medication, is the high rate of noncompliance (24). Single daily doses (pemoline and sustained-release methylphenidate) may enhance compliance, but it is possible that sustained-release methylphenidate may not be as effective as the standard form (25). If the problems occur principally at school, medication may be discontinued on weekends, holidays, and summer vacation.

The most common side effects of stimulant medication are insomnia and decreased appetite, but irritability, weight loss, headache, and abdominal pain may also occur (7). If side effects are severe, the drug may have to be discontinued. A rare but important side effect, which may not remit with discontinuation of medication, is tics. Children who develop tics on stimulants should be *taken off the medication immediately* (7).

Behavioral treatment of Attention Deficit Disorder has focussed principally on helping parents and teachers increase the child's compliance with their requests, increase task completion, and decrease disruptive behavior. As well, some work has been done in teaching children self-control skills (26). There is FIRM EVIDENCE that compliance training is effective (21,27) and SUGGESTIVE EVIDENCE (26) that self-control skills are useful in terms of short-term benefits at home and in the classroom. These results are valid when the treatment is delivered by trained therapists. However, there is NO CLEAR EVIDENCE of the long-term efficacy of behavioral treatments for academic achievement or behavior. The lack of evidence for long-term efficacy of both behavior therapy and medical therapy may be due to the virtual impossibility of long-term research in this area (28) and thus may not reflect the actual inefficacy of the treatments. As well, NO CLEAR EVIDENCE exists of the effectiveness of behavioral treatment when delivered by physicians not specially trained in the field or of treatment delivered in the course of routine office visits. Compliance with the treatment program is also a major problem in determining the effectiveness of behavioral treatment (29).

Perhaps the most important role of the primary physician in helping families with a child who has an Attention Deficit Disorder is as confidant and advisor. Members of a family with a hyperactive child are most likely to have psychological problems themselves. However, this seems to be due to the genetic nature of the disorder and the stress of having a child with a long-term problem rather than the cause of the child's hyperactivity (7). Reassurance that the problem is not the fault of the parents or of the child but is a physical disorder that they can learn to live with is of great help to many families.

Difficult temperament

The management of difficult temperament in children up to 18 months old can consist of reassurance of the parents that the child's behavior is due to normal variations in temperament and not the result of bad parenting; modification of the environment to prevent problems, for instance, child-proofing the home, having a quiet time before bedtime; and parental respites to alleviate their stress.

As previously mentioned, behavior problems in children of this age (and older) have been found to be associated with marital conflict and with parental, especially maternal, depression (7). The direction of causality is not clear and is probably bidirectional; child behavior problems probably both cause and are caused by parental conflict and depression. The focus of treatment, be it the parents' problems or the child's problems, should depend on the relative contribution of each to the family's overall difficulties and the accessibility of treatment.

Unrealistic parental expectations

The main focus of the management of the problem of parents' having unrealistic standards for their child's behavior must be the modification of their standards as well as the improvement of their problem-solving skills. It is necessary but not sufficient to provide such parents with information about what should be expected of children at various ages. Specific suggestions for management of "normal" behavior problems made in the context of an ongoing trusting relationship with the primary care physician are also required. Because of the higher risk of abuse in families with unrealistic expectations for child behavior, close follow-up is advised.

There are a number of popular treatments for behavior problems in children that are touted in the press as being extremely effective and yet scientific support for their effectiveness is lacking. These overlap considerably with cure-alls for learning problems and are reviewed in Chapter 21.

REFERENCES

1. Peterson, R.F. Power, programming, and punishment: Could we by overcontrolling our children? In *Behavior Modification and Families*, Mash, E.J., Hammerlynck, L.A., Handy, L.C., eds. New York: Brunner/Mazel, 1976.
2. Risley, T.R., Clark, H.B., Cataldo, M. Behavioral technology for the normal middle-class family. In *Behavior Modification and Families*, Mash, E.J., Hammerlynck, L.A., Handy, L.C., eds. New York: Brunner/Mazel, 1976.

3. Forehand, R.L., McMahon R.J. *Helping the Noncompliant Child: A Clinician's Guide to Parent Training.* New York: Guilford, 1981.
4. Richman, N., Stevenson, J.E., Graham, P.J. Prevalence of behavior problems in 3-year-old children: An epidemiological study in a London borough. *J. Child. Psychol. Psychiatry* 16:277–287, 1975.
5. Rutter, M., Tizard, J., Whitmore, K. *Education, Health and Behavior.* London: Longman, 1970.
6. Rutter, M. The city and the child. *Am. J. Orthopsychiatry* 51:610–625, 1981.
7. Barkley, R.A. *Hyperactive Children: A Handbook for Diagnosis and Treatment.* New York: Guilford, 1981.
8. American Psychiatric Association. *Diagnostic and Statistical Manual of Mental Disorders,* 3d ed. Washington, D.C.: American Psychiatric Association, 1980.
9. Thomas, A., Chess, S. *Temperament and Development.* New York: Brunner/Mazel, 1977.
10. Offord, D., Waters, B. Socialization and its failure. In *Developmental-Behavioral Pediatrics,* Levine, M.D., Carey, W.B., Crocker, A.C., Gross, R.T., eds. Philadelphia: W.B. Saunders, 1983, pp. 650–682.
11. Robinson, E.A., Eyberg, S.M., Ross, A.W. The standardization of an inventory of child conduct problem behaviors. *J. Clin. Child. Psychol.* 9:22–28, 1980.
12. Eyberg, S.M., Robinson, E.A. Conduct problem behavior: Standardization of a behavioral rating scale with adolescents. *J. Clin. Child Psychol.* 12:347–354, 1983.
13. Griest, D.L., Forehand, R., Wells, K.C., McMahon, R. An examination of differences between nonclinic and behavior problem clinic-referred children and their mothers. *J. Abnorm. Psychol.* 89:497–500, 1980.
14. Carey, W.B. Clinical assessment of behavioral style or temperament. In *Developmental-Behavioral Pediatrics,* Levine, M.D., Carey, W.B., Crocker, A.C., Gross, R.T., eds. Philadelphia: W.B. Saunders, 1983, pp. 922–926.
15. Azar, S.T., Robinson, D.R., Hekimian, E., Twentyman, C.T. Unrealistic expectations and problem solving ability in maltreating and comparison mothers. *J. Consult. Clin. Psychol.* 52:687-691, 1984.
16. Christophersen, E.R. Behavioral pediatrics: An overview. In *Pediatric and Adolescent Behavioral Medicine: Issues in Treatment,* McGrath, P.J., Firestone, P., eds. New York: Springer, 1983.
17. Christophersen, E.R. Incorporating behavioral pediatrics into primary care. *Pediatr. Clin. North Am.* 29:261–296, 1983.
18. Pelham, W.E., Murphy, H.A. Behavioral and pharmacological treatment of attention deficit disorder and conduct disorders. In *Pharmacological and Behavioral Treatment: An Interactive Approach,* Hersen, M., Breuning, S.E., eds. New York: Wiley (in press).
19. Patterson, G.R., Reid, J.B. Intervention for families of aggressive boys: A replication study. *Behav. Res. Ther.* 11:383–394, 1973.
20. York, P., York, D., Wachtel, T. *Toughlove.* New York: Doubleday, 1982.
21. Firestone, P., Kelly, M.J., Goodman, J.T., Davey, J. Differential effects of parent training and stimulant medication with hyperactives. *J. Am. Acad. Child Psychiatr.* 20:135–147, 1981.
22. Gittleman-Klein, R., Abikoff, H., Pollack, E., Klein, D.F., Katz, S., Mattes, J.A. A controlled trial of behavior modification and methylphenidate in hyperactive children. In *Hyperactive Children: The Social Ecology of Identification and Treatment,* Whalen, C., Henker, B., eds. New York: Academic Press, 1980.
23. Barkley, R.A., Cunningham, C.E. Do stimulant drugs improve academic performance of hyperactive children? *Clin. Pediatr.* 17:85–92, 1978.

24. Firestone, P. Factors associated with children's adherence to stimulant medication. *Am. J. Orthopsychiatry* 52:447–457, 1982.
25. Sustained-release methylphenidate. *Medical Let. Drugs Ther.* 26:95-96, 1984.
26. Douglas, V., Parry, P., Marton, P., Garson, C. Assessment of a cognitive training program for hyperactive children. *J. Abnorm. Child Psychol.* 4:389–410, 1976.
27. Mash, E.J., Dalby, T. Behavioral interactions for hyperactivity. In *Hyperactivity in Children: Etiology, Measurement and Treatment Implications*, Trites, R., ed. Baltimore: University Park Press, 1979.
28. Firestone, P., Crowe, D., Goodman, J.T., McGrath, P. Vicissitudes of follow-up studies: Differential effects of parent training and stimulant medication with hyperactives. *Am. J. Orthopsychiatry* 56:184–194, 1986.
29. Firestone, P., Witt, J.E. Characteristics of families completing and prematurely discontinuing a behavioral parent-training program. *J. Pediatr. Psychol.* 7:209–222, 1982.

21

PROBLEMS OF LEARNING

Learning problems cover a wide range of difficulties that have been defined in overlapping and contradictory ways. In this chapter, four problems are considered: mental retardation, specific learning disabilities, communication problems, and learning problems secondary to chronic illness. This arbitrary approach to classification has been taken with the full realization that it does not do justice to the complexities of all the learning problems experienced by children. However, learning problems represent a huge area of study and a thorough discussion of all aspects of learning problems is beyond the scope of this chapter.

The role of the primary care physician in learning problems is in dispute. Some authors (1–3) have outlined a vast array of tests and procedures that the physician can use to diagnose and treat learning problems. We have not taken that approach. The focus of this chapter is on discussion of the assessment and intervention strategies that are appropriate for use by the primary care physician and examination of the indications for referral. In addition, we describe the tools used by specialists in sufficient detail to enable the primary care physician to understand specialists' reports. A final section deals with controversial treatments.

PREVALENCE

The prevalence of learning problems depends on the definition of the term "learning problem." Mental retardation, statistically defined as an IQ at least two standard deviations below the mean on a standard test of intelligence, occurs by definition in 2 to 3% of children (4). Another definition of mental retardation is significantly subaverage general intellectual functioning concurrent with deficits in adaptive behavior and manifested during the developmental period (4).

Definitions of specific learning disabilities vary considerably but generally include the notion of failure in school, in spite of reasonable instruction, combined with average intelligence and no concurrent emotional disturbance. This definition affects prevalence; a learning disability not associated with retardation occurs in approximately 10 to 16% of school-aged children (5).

Communication problems include language disorders, articulation disorders, voice disorders, and stuttering. They occur in 7 to 18% of children (6,7). Learning problems have been estimated to occur in 30 to 40% of children with chronic illness (8,9).

NARROWING DOWN

Mental retardation

About 5% of cases of mental retardation are due to hereditary disorders. Children with inherited causes for retardation often have multiple physical problems that frequently are progressive. Examples include inborn errors of metabolism, such as Tay-Sachs disease, Hurler's syndrome, and phenylketonuria (see Chapter 14).

Approximately one-third of cases of retardation are due to early alterations of embryonic development, including chromosomal changes such as Down's syndrome, and early prenatal influences such as intrauterine infections and use of alcohol and other drugs. These usually result in a relatively stable handicap. A further 11% of mental retardation is the result of problems in the last two trimesters of pregnancy or at birth. These include fetal malnutrition and perinatal difficulties. The handicap usually is not progressive. Acquired childhood diseases or accidents cause approximately 4% of mental retardation, while environmental and behavioral problems such as deprivation, parental psychosis, and childhood mental illness are implicated in another 17%. The cause of almost one-third of cases of mental retardation is unknown or associated with a mixture of possible causes so that a primary cause cannot be discerned (10).

Narrowing down the problem of retardation should always include a careful developmental history. Although the yield of information may be low, a physical examination is also appropriate. Facile reassurance of the parents that everything is all right must be balanced against the negative effects of incorrectly diagnosing mental retardation.

Retardation in newborns Retardation due to hereditary and chromosomal causes is likely to be detected during the newborn period (see Chapter 14). In this age group, unusual but treatable causes of retardation include phenylketonuria and hypothyroidism; screening programs for these are in place in most parts of the developed world. Retardation due to perinatal difficulties may be diagnosed or suspected at this time. Standardized neurological examinations (11) and standardized behavioral assessments (12) have been developed but are not in general clinical use. There is NO CLEAR EVIDENCE that they have predictive value in detecting subsequent learning problems.

Retardation in infants The failure to detect marked hearing impairment in an infant can result in serious developmental delay (see Chapters 3 and 14). *Parents' concerns about their infant's hearing should always be taken seriously.* Untreated hearing problems will lead to major language problems. An important preventable cause of retardation is head trauma (see Chapter 24).

The infant's development should be assessed at each well-baby visit. Formal methods, of which the Denver Developmental Screening Test (13) is the most widely used, or informal methods can be used. Informal methods involve questioning the parents about the child's progress since the last visit and about their concerns, and checking specific milestones. Table 21-1 lists important milestones and the ages by which they should be noted. A suggested advantage of the Denver is that its structured nature ensures that major items are not missed; however, there are several negative aspects to the test as well. The Denver takes about 15 to 20 minutes to administer (A quicker, 5- to 10-minute Denver Prescreening Developmental Questionnaire [14] can be used). It may arouse unnecessary anxiety in parents if their child "fails" an item. A more important disadvantage is that good evidence of the predictive validity of the Denver is seriously lacking. It has very low sensitivity when used in a typical sample of children previously presumed to be developmentally normal (15) and very low specificity when used in a population of rural, disadvantaged children (16). However, other researchers have claimed good predictive validity for the test (17). Informal but careful methods are recommended because of these limitations.

If there is reason for concern, a more detailed assessment is in order, initially by the primary care physician and then by a consultant. The Denver may be of use in these circumstances. Diagnosis can be based only on a very thorough medical examination and an intensive evaluation using diagnostic tests.

Retardation in preschool-aged children Some children will not be suspected of being retarded until the preschool years, when speech and language delays signal a serious problem. The methods of narrowing down the problem are similar to those used in infants. Regular inquiry of the parents about how the child is doing is the recommended strategy. Table 21-2 lists the developmental milestones in this age group. Diagnosis will require consultation with a specialist.

Retardation in school-aged children Although most mentally retarded children are diagnosed before they are of school age, some children with mild retardation are not. Also, there is a need for continually assessing the previously diagnosed child's progress. During the school years, behavior and

Table 21-1. Developmental milestones in infants

Age range (months)	Behavior
0–1	Smiles; reflex head turn; responds to sound; vocalizes
1–4	Lifts chin, chest; holds head erect when held; grasps objects in hand; coos
4–6	Holds head steady; reaches for objects; turns from side to back; rolls over; babbles
6–9	Sits with support; sits alone; smiles at self in mirror; pulls self to stand; stands with help; imitates some sounds; suffers stranger anxiety
9–12	Imitates sounds; says "mamma" or "dadda"; uses pincer grasp; looks for objects; plays peek-a-boo

social problems secondary to retardation may grow to be of more concern than the learning problems. Narrowing down any learning problem in a school-aged child requires consultation (often by telephone) with the child's teacher.

Learning disabilities

The cause of learning disabilities is unknown (5). Some children with learning disabilities have "soft" neurological signs suggestive of neurological damage, but others do not. There is evidence that some cases of learning disability are genetically transmitted. Children with learning disabilities most frequently have a reading disability, but some have a specific spelling, arithmetic, or writing disability. However, there can be considerable variation in the degree of disability even within the same area of disability. The primary care physician should take an active interest in each child's progress in school. Frequently, the family doctor will be the only person outside the school system to whom parents can turn for advice and help with their child's difficulties.

Table 21-2. Developmental milestones in preschool aged children

Age range (months)	Behavior
12–18	Walks alone; can say 5–10 words; points to body parts; uses words to express needs
18–24	Uses 2-word combinations; walks up stairs; points to items when named; follows simple commands
24–36	Uses 3- to 4-word sentences; understands "in", "on", "under"; can count 3–5 objects; says own name, age, and sex; can dress with help
36–48	Uses 4- to 5-word sentences; follows 2-part commands; counts 4–6 objects; uses past tense

Whereas diagnosis of mental retardation will almost always be made by the preschool years, most learning disabilities will be diagnosed during the school years. When parents of a preschool-aged child are concerned about their child's learning, the problems are almost always due to a communication disorder. These are discussed below. Parents whose preschool-aged children are communicating well but do not yet read or write should be reassured that children vary widely in the development of skills such as reading and writing, and that early development does not presage later accomplishment.

Communication disorders

Children with orofacial abnormalities, for example, cleft palate, have a high rate of articulation, voice, and resonance problems that are usually detected at birth or shortly afterward and are treated by a specialty team in a tertiary care facility. Children with a developmental language delay can be detected during routine visits to the primary care physician by questioning the parents about what the child says. Tables 21-1 and 21-2 describe the speech and language milestones that should be assessed. Speech dysfluencies (repetitions or hesitations) are developmentally normal in the 2- to 3-year-old and, in most instances, will spontaneously remit if they are ignored. Stuttering should be considered a possibility only if there is pervasive and persistent repetition of entire words or sounds that interfere with communication and are stressful to the *child*. Articulation difficulties (mispronunciation of sounds) are normal in preschool-aged children, and unless the child's speech is almost unintelligible, there is NO CLEAR EVIDENCE that formal assessment prior to kindergarten is beneficial. Voice problems are manifested as unusual voice quality such as hoarseness or high pitch at any age.

Learning problems in chronic illness

The learning problems of children with chronic illness may result from the illness itself (direct effects of the illness on the central nervous system, fatigue and stress, drugs used to treat the illness) or because of interruptions in the child's school attendance. Except for children with central nervous system involvement, there is NO CLEAR EVIDENCE why so many children with chronic illness have learning problems (7,8). Some information is available about the effects of specific illnesses or treatments:

1. A small but significant number of asthmatic children treated with theophylline develop learning problems that remit when theophylline is replaced with another drug (18). In some cases, the physician and family are confronted with a paradoxical situation: Aggressive pharmacotherapy may result in learning problems because of the

side effects of the theophylline, but failure to treat the asthma aggressively may result in problems in school because of poor attendance.

2. Children with cancer who have been treated by central nervous system irradiation (FIRM EVIDENCE) or intrathecal methotrexate (SUGGESTIVE EVIDENCE) experience a general lowering of cognitive ability and performance. No such effect has been reported from systemically administered anticancer drugs (19,20).
3. Children whose diabetes is not well controlled are likely to learn less efficiently (SUGGESTIVE EVIDENCE) (8).
4. Children who have had chronic otitis media and resultant mild conductive hearing loss (21) may be at greater risk for language difficulties (SUGGESTIVE EVIDENCE).
5. Children with cyanotic congenital heart disease may show general decrements in learning, which may respond to appropriate surgery (SUGGESTIVE EVIDENCE) (8).
6. Children who are receiving antiepileptic drugs, particularly phenobarbital and perhaps phenytoin, may suffer from inattention as a side effect of their medication (SUGGESTIVE EVIDENCE) (22,23).

Narrowing down a learning problem associated with chronic illness will include the same tests used to determine retardation and learning disabilities, but it does require a consultant who is familiar with the specific problems associated with a particular child's illness.

DIAGNOSIS OF LEARNING PROBLEMS

The diagnosis of all types of learning problems is usually made by a consultant specialist or a team of consultants, including educational and developmental psychologists, developmental pediatricians, and speech and language pathologists. Individually administered psychological tests measuring both general ability or intelligence and specific abilities are the primary tools used for determining retardation and evaluating learning disabilities. Speech and language tests are used to measure communication disorders. Standardized and diagnostic achievement measures are used to determine what a child has learned. Specific abilities tests are used to narrow down the precise nature of the problem.

The administration and interpretation of tests should be carried out by qualified personnel. Intelligence and other abilities testing should be done by or directly supervised by a registered or licensed psychologist, who generally possesses a doctorate in clinical, developmental, or educational psychology. Achievement tests and screening tests may be given by teachers trained in their administration and interpretation. If the problem is one of speech and language, a speech and language pathologist or therapist may be very helpful. Speech and language specialists are usually trained at the master's level and are certified by the national speech and language association. Test results must be interpreted in light of prior test data, the child's history, cultural background, primary language, physical handicap, motivation, ability to concentrate, and physical and emotional state during testing. The major task a consultant faces in diagnosis is to distinguish between learning disabilities and mental retardation, and among emotional, language, or attention deficit disorders, and to provide specific information about the educational management and prognosis. It is not unusual for such an assessment to take 6 to 10 hours over several sessions.

Table 21-3 summarizes the most common tests used in assessing children with learning problems. This summary is, of necessity, cursory. In particular, the very large number of standardized educational tests have not been included. Consultation with a trusted specialist will be necessary for tests not included in the table. As well, the test manuals, standard textbooks (24,25), or the *Mental Measurements Yearbook* (26) can be consulted for more detailed descriptions of each test. The tests are listed in alphabetical order and are designated as *General* tests, which measure global intelligence or cognitive ability; *Specific* tests, which measure individual abilities; and *Achievement* tests, which measure what the child has learned in specific areas.

A good test in the hands of a qualified examiner is necessary for an appropriate assessment. Although primary care physicians will not be administering the tests or directly interpreting results, it is important that they know how good a test is and what it is supposed to measure. Usually, exact scores will not be given in psychological reports because of the lack of precision of the results and the danger of overinterpretation of such scores. However, ranges or description of the scores are usually provided.

ASSISTANCE WITH LEARNING PROBLEMS

Unfortunately, most forms of learning problems are not curable. However, the primary care physician has several major roles in the treatment of the problems faced by these children and their families:

1. Detection and treatment (when possible) of the medical aspects of learning problems.
2. Provision of balanced therapeutic optimism and ongoing emotional support.
3. Referrals to consultants and coordination and interpretation of conflicting or confusing reports.
4. Advocacy for appropriate educational intervention.
5. Recognition and assistance when secondary problems arise, for example, behavior problems or parental stress.

Table 21-3. Common tests used in learning problems

Test:	American Association on Mental Deficiency Adaptive Behavior Scale (ABS) (27).
Description:	There are two version of the Scale, one for institutionalized children and one for children in public schools. Both measure adaptive behavior in retarded children.
Type:	Specific.
Evaluation:	Useful measure of adaptive and maladaptive behavior in school children.
Test:	Ammons Quick Test (28).
Description:	Nonverbal multiple choice test: measures receptive vocabulary from age 2 to adult, yielding mental age or IQ scores; takes 3 to 10 minutes.
Evaluation:	This is not an intelligence test. A useful vocabulary test.
Test:	Balthazar Scales of Adaptive Behavior (29).
Description:	Assesses functional independence and social adaptation in the severely and profoundly retarded.
Type:	Specific.
Evaluation:	Helpful for measuring functioning in this group of children.
Test:	Bayley Scales of Infant Development (30).
Description:	Individually administered by a psychologist for infants 2 months to 2½ years old. Yields a Mental Developmental Index and a Psychomotor Developmental Index, each of which has a mean of 100 and a standard deviation of 16.
Type:	General, Specific.
Evaluation:	The best measure of infant development.
Test:	Bender Visual Motor Gestalt Test (BVMGT) (31).
Description:	Child is asked to copy geometric designs. Yields developmental scores with a mean of 100 and a standard deviation of 15.
Type:	Specific.
Evaluation:	Useful as an adjunctive test in evaluating visual motor abilities.
Test:	Frostig Developmental Test of Visual Perception (DTVP) (32).
Description:	Nonverbal test of visual perception for children ages 3 to 9 years.
Type:	Specific.
Evaluation:	A measure of visual perception, not a reading readiness test. Remediation should not be based on subtest deficits.
Test:	Halstead Neuropsychological Test Battery for Children (33).
Description:	The Reitan-Indiana equivalent for children aged 9-14 years.
Type:	General, Specific.
Evaluation:	The most widely used and respected battery for evaluating children of this age with suspected brain damage. Usually accompanied by WISC-R (see below).
Test:	Illinois Test of Psycholinguistic Abilities, Revised Edition (ITPA) (34).
Description:	A measure of twelve verbal skills in children aged 2 years, 4 months to 10 years, 3 months. Scaled scores have a mean of 36 and a standard deviation of 6; psycholinguistic age can be computed.
Type:	General, Specific.
Evaluation:	Subtests do not measure different abilities but measure general verbal ability. Not a very useful test for determining type of learning disability.
Test:	Kaufman Assessment Battery for Children (K-ABC) (35).
Description:	Individually administered by psychologist for children aged 2½ to 12½ years. There are sixteen subtests, ten of which are designed to assess mental processing and six of which are achievement tests.
Type:	General, Specific.
Evaluation:	Well-constructed, relatively new test that may be useful in determining strengths and deficiencies in learning disabilities.
Test:	Leiter International Performance Scale (36).
Description:	Measure intelligence from 2 years to adult by nonverbal methods.

Table 21-3. Common tests used in learning problems   (*cont'd.*)

Type:	General.
Evaluation:	Norms outdated; standardization poor but may be helpful as a supplementary test in children with verbal problems.
Test:	Luria-Nebraska Neuropsychological Battery—Children's Revision (37).
Description:	A neuropsychological battery for use in children age 8 to 12 years, based on an adult battery.
Type:	General, Specific.
Evaluation:	Relatively new battery that is not yet firmly established. For children with suspected brain damage.
Test:	McCarthy Scales of Children's Abilities (38).
Description:	Individually administered by psychologist for children 2½ to 8½ years. Eighteen tests grouped into six scales. Provides a General Cognitive Index with a median of 100 and a standard deviation of 16.
Type:	General, Specific.
Evaluation:	Good tests. May be particularly useful for assessing specific abilities in preschool-aged children.
Test:	Metropolitan Achievement Test, Fifth Edition (39).
Description:	Group test for children from kindergarten through grade 12 that measures achievement in language, mathematics, reading, science, and social studies.
Type:	Achievement.
Evaluation:	Excellent achievement test that provides and understanding of how a child functions under classroom like conditions.
Test:	Otis-Lennon Mental Ability Test (40).
Description:	Group test intended to measure global intelligence.
Type:	General.
Evaluation:	Useful only as a very rough screening test.
Test:	Peabody Individual Achievement Test (PIAT) (41).
Description:	Individually administred test measuring mathematics, reading recognition, reading comprehension, spelling, and general information. All tests are untimed.
Type:	Achievement.
Evaluation:	A brief, limited test of school achievement.
Test:	Peabody Picture Vocualary Test—Revised (PPVT-R) (42).
Description:	Nonverbal multiple-choice test of receptive vocabulary for ages 2½ years to adult. Yields a standard score with a mean of 100 and a standard deviation of 15.
Type:	Specific.
Evaluation:	This is not an intelligence test. A useful receptive vocabulary test, especially for children with expressive difficulties.
Test:	Raven's Progressive Matricies (43).
Description:	Test of nonverbal reasoning using figure recognition for ages 6 years to adult.
Type:	General.
Evaluation:	No North American norms. Measures only one element of reasoning; may be less culturally biased than some other tests.
Test:	Reitan-Indiana Neuropsychological Test Battery (44).
Description:	Neuropsychological battery for children aged 5 to 8 years, modeled on the well-stablished adult battery.
Type:	General, Specific.
Evaluation:	Most widely used and respected battery to evaluate children of this age with suspected brain damage. Usually accompanied by WISC-R or WPPSI (see below).

Table 21-3. Common tests used in learning problems   (*cont'd.*)

Test:	Slosson Intelligence Test for Children and Adults (45).
Description:	For age 5 months to 22 years. Takes 10 to 30 minutes to administer.
Type:	General.
Evaluation:	Poorly standardized. Useful only as a screening instrument.
Test:	Stanford Achievement Test, Seventh Edition (SAT) (46).
Description:	Comprehensive set of achievement tests for children from grade 1 to 12. Covers reading, mathematics, spelling, science, and social studies. Can be administered to a group or individually.
Type:	Achievement.
Evaluation:	A well constructed test covering a wide range of school subjects. The total battery can take more than 6 hours to administer.
Test:	Stanford-Binet, Fourth Edition (47).
Description:	Individually administered for individuals from 2 to adult. Provides scores of verbal reasoning, quantitative reasoning, abstract/visual reasoning, and short-term memory, and a composite score.
Type:	General, Specific.
Evaluation:	The first IQ test, now thoroughly updated. Excellent test; usually used for preschool-aged children.
Test:	Vineland Adaptive Behavior Scales [replaces the Vineland Social Maturity Scale] (48).
Description:	Three different forms measure communication skill, daily living skills, and socialization and motor skills in children from birth to 19 years.
Type:	Specific.
Evaluation:	Well-validated set of scales to measure adaptive skills.
Test:	Wechsler Intelligence Scale for Children—Revised (WISC-R) (49).
Description:	Intelligence test for children aged 6 to 16 years, 11 months. Yields verbal, performance, and full-scale IQ with a mean of 100 and a standard deviation of 15.
Type:	General, Specific.
Evaluation:	Excellent test, the standard against which all others are evaluated.
Test:	Wechsler Preschool and Primary Scale of Intelligence (WPPSI) (50).
Description:	Downward extension of WISC-R for children aged 4 to 6½ years. Six verbal subtests and five performance subtests generate a verbal scale, a performance scale, and a full-scale IQ. Average IQ is 100, with a standard deviation of 15.
Type:	General, Specific.
Evaluation:	Excellent.
Test:	Wepman Auditory Discrimination Test (ADT) (51).
Description:	Forty word pairs are used to assess auditory discrimination.
Type:	Specific.
Evaluation:	Should be used only as a rough screening instrument.
Test:	Wide Range Achievement Test, 1984 revision (WRAT) (52).
Description:	Achievement test that measures aspects of reading, spelling, and arithmetic.
Type:	Achievement.
Evaluation:	Newly revised version is methodologically sound and promises to be excellent; earlier versions were less well constructed but widely used.
Test:	Woodcock-Johnson Psycho-Educational Battery (53).
Description:	Contains 27 tests covering intellectual ability, achievement, and interests. Can yield a standard score with a mean of 100 and a standard deviation of 15.
Type:	General, Specific, Achievement.
Evaluation:	Comprehensive battery not widely enough used to determine how useful it will be.

There is NO CLEAR EVIDENCE to support the use of one specific type of educational setting over another, such as integrated as opposed to specialty classes or schools for retarded children, or resource withdrawal as opposed to special classes for the learning disabled. However, proper placement is most likely to allow development of the abilities that a child already has, enhance the child's self-esteem, and increase the parents' and teachers' ability to cope. There is FIRM EVIDENCE (54) that remedial teaching can effectively help children with reading disabilities and that comprehensive, individualized education can help preschool-aged, economically deprived, minority children achieve in subsequent years of school (55). There is NO CLEAR EVIDENCE that therapy for language delay, articulation difficulties, or voice disorders is effective (7). However, there is evidence that children with these problems are at higher risk for behavior or emotional problems (7) and they will probably need assistance. There is FIRM EVIDENCE that treatment of established stutterers by trained therapists using prolonged speech or precision fluency shaping is efficacious (56).

Controversial treatments

There is NO CLEAR EVIDENCE that any of the simplistic treatments that promise cures for learning problems, such as patterning, the Feingold diet, treatment of hypoglycemia or reduction of amount of sugar consumed, treatment of brain allergy, megavitamins, vitamins plus minerals, sensory integrative therapy, vestibular drugs, and visual training, are in any way helpful.

Table 21-4 details the current status of these controversial treatments. It is clear that the extraordinary claims made for them are not warranted. Also, some of the treatments may be harmful because they raise false hopes and expectations, drain families financially or emotionally, and delay appropriate treatment. In some cases, excessive doses of vitamins or lengthy hours of repetitive training may physically harm the child.

Several authors have suggested that the lead levels commonly found in the blood of urban children are responsible for their learning problems (76). There is NO CLEAR EVIDENCE (77) of such a relationship. Whether other minerals or trace elements contribute to learning disabilities is unclear (78). There is NO CLEAR EVIDENCE of the efficacy of any treatment based on the administration of minerals or trace elements.

There is FIRM EVIDENCE for an immediate relationship between eating breakfast and academic performance (79,80), but no sound, long-term data exist. Physicians should encourage their patients to eat breakfast and should support school breakfast programs.

Table 21-4. Controversial treatments for learning problems

	Proponent	Evaluation (NO CLEAR EVIDENCE in all cases)
Patterning	Doman-Delacato (57)	Useless; very costly in terms of time invested; may be harmful (58)
Feingold diet	Feingold (59)	FIRM EVIDENCE that this does not help (61)
Elimination of sugar from the diet	Various	FIRM EVIDENCE of no effect (61)
Brain allergy	Wunderlich (62)	Treatment with steroids probably dangerous
Megavitamin therapy	Orthomolecular psychiatrists/ psychologists	Excessive vitamin A can cause brain edema; excessive vitamin C may contribute to kidney stones (63)
Megavitamins & mineral therapy	Harrell et al. (64)	FIRM EVIDENCE that this does not help (65)
Sensory integration therapy	Ayres (66)	SUGGESTIVE EVIDENCE that this does not work (67); questionable premise (68)
Vestibular drug	Levinson (69, 70)	Questionable premise (68)
Visual training	"developmental" optometrists	Often expensive; questionable premise (71–73)
Listening training	Tomatis (74)	Expensive, questionable premise. FIRM EVIDENCE (75) that this does not help.

REFERENCES

1. Levine, M.D., Brooks, R., Shonkoff, J.P. *A Pediatric Approach to Learning Disorders*. New York: John Wiley, 1980.
2. Accardo, P.J., Capute, A.J. *The Pediatrician and the Developmentally Delayed Child: A Clinical Textbook on Mental Retardation*. Baltimore: University Park Press, 1979.
3. Illingworth, R.S. *The Development of the Infant and Young Child: Normal and Abnormal*. New York: Churchill Livingstone, 1974.
4. Grossman, H.J., ed. *Classification in Mental Retardation*. Washington, D.C.: American Association on Mental Deficiency, 1983.
5. Ferguson, H.B., Mamen, M. Learning disabilities: Etiology, diagnosis and management. *Psychiatric Clinics of North America* 8:703–720, 1985.
6. Bax, M., Hart, M. Health needs of preschool children. *Arch. Dis. Child.* 51:848–852, 1976.
7. Baker, L., Cantwell, D.P. Primary prevention of the psychiatric consequences of childhood communication disorders. *J. Prev. Psychiatr.* 2:75–79, 1985.
8. Schlieper, A. Chronic illness and school achievement. *Dev. Med. Child Neurol.* 27:75–79, 1985.
9. Fowler, M.G., Johnson, M.P., Atkinson, S.S. School achievement and absence in children with chronic health conditions. *J. Pediatr.* 106:683–687, 1985.
10. Crocker, A.C., Nelson, R.P. Mental retardation. In *Developmental-Behavioral Pediatrics*, Levine, M.D., Carey, W.B., Crocker, A.C., Gross, R.T., eds. Philadelphia: W.B. Saunders, 1983.
11. Prechtl, H.F.R., Beintema, J. *The Neurological Examination of the Full-term Newborn Infant*. Clinics in Developmental Medicine, No. 28. London: Spastics International Medical Publications, 1968.

12. Brazelton, T.B. *Neonatal Behavioral Assessment Scale*, 2d ed. Clinics in Developmental Medicine, No. 88. London: Spastics International Medical Publications, 1984.
13. Frankenburg, W.K., Dodds, J.B. The Denver developmental screening test. *J. Pediatr.* 71:181, 1967.
14. Frankenburg, W.K., van Doorninck, W.J., Liddell, T.N., Dick, N.P. The Denver prescreening developmental questionnaire. *Pediatrics* 57:744–753, 1976.
15. Cadman, D., Chambers, L.W., Walter, S.D., Feldman, W., Smith, K., Ferguson, R. The usefulness of the Denver Developmental Screening Test to predict kindergarten problems in a general community. *Am. J. Public Health* 74:1093–1097, 1984.
16. Harper, D., Wacker, D.P. The efficiency of the Denver Developmental Screening Test with rural disadvantaged preschool children. *J. Pediatr. Psychol.* 8:273–283, 1983.
17. Sturner, R.A., Green, J.A., Funk, S.G. Preschool Denver Developmental Screening Test as a predictor of later school problems. *J. Pediatr.* 107:615–621, 1985.
18. Furukawa, C.T., Shapiro, G.G., DuHamel, T., Weimer, L., Pierson, W.E., Bierman, C.W. Learning and behaviour problems associated with theophylline therapy. *Lancet* 1:621, 1984.
19. Copeland, D.R., Fletcher, J.M., Pfefferbaum-Levine, B., Jaffe, N., Reid, H., Maor, M. Neuropsychological sequelae of childhood cancer in long-term survivors. *Pediatrics* 75:745–753, 1985.
20. Lansky, S.B., Cairns, G.F., Cairns, N.U., Stephenson, L., Lansky, L.L., Garin, G. Central nervous system prophylaxis. *Am. J. Pediatr. Hematol. Oncol.* 6:183–190, 1984.
21. Schlieper, A., Kisilevsky, H., Mattingly, S., Yorke, L. Mild conductive hearing loss and language development: A one year follow-up study. *Developmental and Behavioral Pediatrics*, 6:65–68, 1985.
22. Trimble, M. Anticonvulsant drugs, behavior and cognitive abilities. *Curr. Dev. Psychopharmacol.* 6:65–91, 1981.
23. American Academy of Pediatrics, Behavioral and cognitive effects of anticonvulsant therapy. *Pediatrics* 76:644–647, 1985.
24. Sattler, J.M. *Assessment of Children's Intelligence and Special Abilities*, 2d ed. Toronto: Allyn & Bacon, 1982.
25. Anastasi, A. *Psychological Testing*, 5th ed. New York: Macmillan, 1982.
26. Buros, O.K., ed. *The Eighth Mental Measurements Yearbook*. Highland Park, N.J.: Gryphon Press, 1978.
27. American Association on Mental Deficiency. *Adaptive Behavior Scales*. Washington: American Association on Mental Deficiency, 1974.
28. Ammons, R.B., Ammons, C.H. The quick test (QT): Provisional manual. *Psychol. Rep.* 11:111–162, 1962.
29. Balthazar, E.E. *Balthazar Scales of Adaptive Behavior*. Palo Alto, Calif.: Consulting Psychologists Press, 1976.
30. Bayley, N. *Bayley Scales of Infant Development: Birth to Two Years*. New York: Psychological Corporation, 1969.
31. Bender, L.A. *Manual for Instruction and Test Cards for Visual Motor Gestalt Test*. New York: American Orthopsychiatric Association, 1946.
32. Frostig, M., Maslow, P., Lefever, D.W., Whittlesey, J.R.B. The Marianne Frostig Developmental Test of Visual Perception, 1963 standardization. *Percept. Mot. Skills* 19:463–499, 1964.
33. Reitan, R. Manual for administration of neuropsychological test batteries for adults and children. Author, 1969.

34. Kirk, S.A., McCarthy, J.J., Kirtk, W. *The Illinois Test of Psycholinguistic Abilities*. Urbana: University of Illinois Press, 1968.

35. Kaufman, A., Kaufman, N. *The Kaufman Assessment Battery for Children*. Circle Pines, Minn.: American Guidance Service, 1983.

36. Arthur, G. The Arthur adaptation of the Leiter International Performance Scale. *J. Clin. Psychol.* 5:345–349, 1949.

37. Golden, C.J., Hammeke, T., Purisch A. *The Luria-Nebraska Battery Manual*. Los Angeles: Western Psychological Services, 1980.

38. McCarthy, D.A. *Manual for the McCarthy Scales of Children's Abilities*. New York: Psychological Corporation, 1972.

39. Balow, I.H., Farr, R., Hogan, T.P., Prescott, G.A. *Metropolitan Achievement Test*, 5th ed. New York: Psychological Corporation, 1978.

40. Otis, A.S., Lennon, R.T. *Otis-Lennon Mental Ability Test: Manual for Administration*. New York: Harcourt Brace Jovanovich, 1967.

41. Dunn, L.M., Markwardt, F.C., Jr. *Peabody Individual Achievement Test*. Circle Pines, Minn.: American Guidance Service, 1970.

42. Dunn, L.M., Dunn, L.M. *Peabody Picture Vocabulary Test—Revised*. Circle Pines, Minn.: American Guidance Service, 1981.

43. Raven, J.C. *Progressive Matrices*. London: Lewis, 1938.

44. Reitan, R.M., Davison, L.A., eds. *Clinical Neuropsychology: Current Status and Applications*. Washington, D.C.: V.H. Winston & Sons, 1974.

45. Slosson, R.L. *Slosson Intelligence Test for Children and Adults*. New York: Slosson Educational Publications, 1963.

46. Madden, R., Gardner, E.F., Rudman, H.C., Karlsen, B., Merwin, J.C. *Stanford Achievement Test*, 7th ed. New York: Psychological Corporation, 1982.

47. Thorndike, R.L., Hagen, E.P., Sattler, J.M. *Stanford Binet Intelligent Scale*, 4th ed. Chicago: Riverside Publishing Co. 1986.

48. Sparrow, S., Balla, D.A., Cicchetti, D.V. *Vineland Adaptive Behavior Scales*. Circle Pines, Minn.: American Guidance Services, 1984.

49. Wechsler, D. *Manual for the Wechsler Intelligence Scale for Children—Revised*. New York: Psychological Corporation, 1974.

50. Wechsler, D. *Manual for the Wechsler Preschool and Primary Scale of Intelligence*. New York: Psychological Corporation, 1967.

51. Wepman, J.M. *The Auditory Discrimination Test*. Chicago: Language Research, 1973.

52. Jastak, S., Wilkinson, G.S. *Wide Range Achievement Test Administration Manual*, rev. ed. Wilmington, Del.: Jastak Associates, 1984.

53. Woodcock, R.W. *Woodcock-Johnson Psycho-Educational Battery: Technical Report*. Boston: Teaching Resources, 1977.

54. Gittleman, R., Finegold, J. Children with reading disorders—a. Efficacy of reading remediation. *J. Child Psychol. Psychiatr.* 24:167–191, 1983.

55. Sparrow, S.S., Blachman, B.A., Chauncey, S. Diagnostic and prescriptive intervention in primary school education. *Am. J. Orthopsychiatry* 53:721–729, 1983.

56. Andrews, G., Craig, A., Feyer, A.M., Hoddinott, S., Howie, P., Neilson, M. Stuttering: A review of research findings and theories circa 1982. *J. Speech Hear. Disord.* 48:226–246, 1983.

57. Delacato, C.H. *The Diagnosis and Treatment of Speech and Reading Problems*. Springfield, Ill.: Charles C Thomas, 1963.

58. American Academy of Cerebral Palsy, American Academy of Neurology, American Academy of Pediatrics, American Academy of Physical and Rehabilitation Medicine, American Academy of Orthopedics; Canadian Association for Children with Learning Disabilities, Canadian Association for Retarded Children;

National Association for Retarded Children (U.S.A.). The Doman-Delacato treatment of neurologically handicapped children. *Neurology* 18:1214–1216, 1968.

59. Feingold, B. *Why Is Your Child Hyperactive?* New York: Random House, 1975.
60. Harley, J.P., Ray, R.S. Tomasi, L., Eichman, P.L., Chun, R., Cleeland, C.S., Traisman, E. Hyperkinesis and food additives: Testing the Feingold hypothesis. *Pediatrics* 61:818–828, 1978.
61. Wolraich, M., Milich, R., Stumbo, P., Schultz, F. Effects of sucrose ingestion on the behavior of hyperactive boys. *J. Pediatr.* 106:675–682, 1985.
62. Wunderlich, R.C. *Allergy, Brains and Children Coping.* St. Petersburg, Fla.: Johnny Reads, 1973.
63. American Academy of Pediatrics Committee on Nutrition. Megavitamin therapy for childhood psychoses and learning disabilities. *Pediatrics* 58:910–912, 1976.
64. Harrell, R.F., Capp, R.H., Davis, D.R., Peerless, J., Ravitz, L.R. Can nutritional supplements help mentally retarded children? An exploratory study. *Proc. Nat. Acad. Sci. U.S.A.* 78:574–578, 1981.
65. Weathers, C. Effects of nutritional supplementation on IQ and certain other variables associated with Down syndrome. *Am. J. Ment. Defic.* 88:214–217, 1983.
66. Ayres, J. *Sensory Integration and Learning Disorders.* Los Angeles: Western Psychological Services, 1972.
67. Carte, E., Morrison, D., Sublett, J., Uemura, A., Setrakian, W. Sensory integration therapy: A trial of a specific neurodevelopmental therapy for the remediation of learning disabilities. *Developmental and Behavioral Pediatrics* 5:189–194, 1984.
68. Polatajko, H.J. A critical look at vestibular dysfunction in learning disabled children. *Dev. Med. Child. Neurol.* 27:283–292, 1985.
69. Levinson, H.N. *A Solution to the Riddle Dyslexia.* New York: Springer Verlag, 1980.
70. Levinson, H.N. *Smart But Feeling Dumb.* New York: Warner Books, 1985.
71. American Academy of Pediatrics, American Academy of Ophthalmology, American Association for Pediatric Ophthalmology and Strabismus: Joint policy statement: Learning disabilities, dyslexia, and vision. January/February 1984.
72. Mann, L. Review of the Marianne Frostig Developmental Test of Visual Perception. In *The Seventh Mental Measurements Yearbook*, Buros, O.K., ed. Highland Park, N.J.: Gryphon Press, 1972, p. 1274–1276.
73. Metzger, R.L., Werner, D.B. Use of visual training for reading disabilities: A review. *Pediatrics* 73:824–829, 1984.
74. Tomatis, A. *Education and dyslexia.* France-Quebec Les Editions, 1978.
75. Kershner, J.R., Cummings, R.L., Clarke, K.A. *Two year evaluation of the Tomatis Listening Training Programme.* Toronto, Ontario: Institute for Studies in Education, 1986.
76. Needleman, H.L., Gunnoe, C., Leviton, A., Reed, R., Peresie, H., Maher, C., Barrett, B.S. Deficits in psychologic and classroom performance of children with elevated dentine lead levels. *N. Engl. J. Med.* 300:689–695, 1979.
77. Smith, M., Delves, T., Lansdown, R. Clayton, B., Graham, P. The effects of lead exposure on urban children: The institute of Child Health/Southampton Study. *Dev. Med. Child Neurol.* (suppl. 47):1–54, 1983.
78. Rimland, B., Larson, G.E. Hair mineral analysis and behavior: An analysis of the literature. *J. Learn. Dis.* 16:279–285, 1983.
79. Conners, C.K., Blouin, A.G. Nutritional effects on behavior of children. *J. Psychiatr. Res.* 17:193–201, 1983.
80. Pollitt, E., Gersovitz, M., Garguilo, M. Educational benefits of the United States school feeding program: A critical review of the literature. *Am. J. Public Health* 68:477–481, 1978.

22

ACHES AND PAINS

Pain is an ubiquitous symptom that can occur in almost any part of the body and can indicate a wide variety of problems. This chapter focusses on benign, recurrent pain problems that are common in children: headache, stomachache, "colic," chest pain, and limb pain. Also, chronic pain syndrome, which constitutes failure to cope with pain, is examined. Colic is included in this chapter even though we have no sure way of determining that babies with colic are in pain.

Many other types of pain are covered in specific chapters: recurrent and acute ear pain in Chapter 3; acute abdominal pain in Chapter 5; pain on urination in Chapter 10; eye pain in Chapter 13; and pain due to injury in Chapter 24. Back pain, while common in adults, is relatively rare in children and adolescents (1) and is not covered here. Postoperative pain is usually not handled by primary care physicians and consequently is not reviewed.

PREVALENCE

The prevalence of recurrent headache, including migraine, in children aged 7 to 15 years has been estimated to be approximately 11%; migraine alone was found to occur in 4% of children (2). Other estimates of prevalence have been higher (3,4), ranging up to 26%.

Recurrent abdominal pain severe enough to interfere with activities occurs in approximately 10 to 15% of children (5). Colic, signaled by the unrelenting crying of young infants for more than 3 hours per day, 3 days or more per week, lasting more than 3 weeks, and for no known reason, has been estimated to occur in about 25% of babies (6).

Chest pain has become a major reason for the referral of children to pediatric cardiology clinics in the United States (7); it accounts for 650,000 patient visits annually for 10- to 21-year-olds (8). The actual prevalence of chest pain is unknown. Limb pain occurs in 4 to 18% of children (9). The prevalence of chronic benign pain syndrome is unknown but is not high.

195

HEADACHE

Narrowing down and diagnosis

The principal task in narrowing down the problem of recurrent headache is to distinguish headache as a symptom of underlying systemic, head, face, neck, or central nervous system pathology from benign headache. The most important tools for making this distinction are a careful history and a thorough physical examination. Table 22-1 outlines the aspects of the history that are important, and Table 22-2 lists those items that should be checked routinely in the physical examination. Routine laboratory tests should not be done — however, specific symptoms should trigger further laboratory investigations.

Once pathological headache is ruled out, benign headache can be further narrowed down to migraine and its variants, muscle contraction headache, and various types of psychogenic headache. Migraine includes common migraine, which is usually bilateral and is not preceded by a prodrome; classical migraine, which is usually unilateral and is preceded by a prodrome; cluster

Table 22-1. Narrowing down the problem of recurrent headache from the patient's history

	Suspect migraine	Suspect muscle contraction	Suspect pathological headache
Family history of migraine	X		
Completely normal physical examination	X	X	
Pain getting worse			X
Headaches last 2–3 hours	X		
1/2-hour prodrome	X		
Nausea or vomiting	X		X
History of motion sickness, breath-holding spells, or syncope	X		
Constant pain		X	X
Bandlike pressure		X	
Attacks related to "stress"		X	
Intellectual decline			X
Personality change			X
Pain in face			X
Waking at night with pain			X
Motor or perceptual difficulties during pain-free intervals			X
Changes in fundi			X
Localizing central nervous system findings			X

Table 22-2. Physical examination for head-ache

1. Height
2. Weight
3. Head circumference
4. Blood pressure
5. Examination of fundi
6. Percussion of sinuses
7. Listening for bruits
8. Examination of skin for neurocutaneous stigmata
9. Complete neurological examination

headaches and the complicated migraines including ophthalmoplegic, hemiplegic, confusional, basilar artery, and Alice-in-Wonderland migraine, which have as their main feature focal neurologic symptoms. Detailed descriptions of these variants of migraine, which are usually treated by a specialist, are available in several recent reviews (10–12). A variant of migraine frequently occurs in the months following head trauma.

Muscle contraction headaches are not paroxysmal and are thought to be due to prolonged muscle tension in the head and neck. They are usually reported to arise late in the day in response to that day's stress. Some children with severe migraine also have muscle contraction headaches between bouts of migraine (mixed headache).

Psychogenic headache usually refers to a persistent and intractable headache of the muscle contraction type. Psychogenic headache can arise from:

1. avoidance or escape from unpleasant events;
2. direct reward for pain behavior (e.g., a parent's comforting);
3. anxiety, especially performance anxiety;
4. depression; and
5. psychosis (12).

Psychogenic pain accompanied by major disruptions in school attendance is discussed in more detail in the section on chronic pain syndrome below.

Management of headache

The management of pathological headache depends on the nature of the problem and is best handled by a consultant. The management of benign headache begins with a complete history and physical examination, which generally are reassuring to the child and family.

The behavioral and medical treatment of migraine can be palliative, prophylactic, or abortive. Palliative behavioral treatment consists of napping or resting at the first sign of an attack (NO CLEAR EVIDENCE). There is NO CLEAR EVIDENCE, because of the lack of research, that palliative medication taken at the first sign of an attack (ASA, acetaminophen, or Fiorinal) is effective.

Prophylactic medication is indicated when the headaches are frequent enough and severe enough to seriously interfere with the child's activities. Propranalol (14,15), which is approved for this purpose, should be prescribed at a dosage of 1 mg/kg/day in two divided doses (NO CLEAR EVIDENCE). Amitriptyline (16) can be prescribed at a dosage of 1 mg/kg/day in two divided doses (NO CLEAR EVIDENCE). Calcium-entry blockers have been suggested as a treatment but their use has not yet been adequately assessed (17). Prophylactic psychological interventions include relaxation training (18–19) and cognitive therapy (18) (SUGGESTIVE EVIDENCE). Unfortunately, these require the services of specially trained professionals.

Muscle contraction headaches can be symptomatically treated with analgesics and heat (NO CLEAR EVIDENCE) or with relaxation training (SUGGESTIVE EVIDENCE) (19).

The treatment of psychogenic headaches must be aimed at ameliorating the cause. In some cases, such as headaches caused by a stressful school-bus ride, environmental manipulation may be effective. Brief, informal counseling may also be helpful. Cases of psychogenic headache that do not respond quickly to simple interventions should be referred to a consultant.

ABDOMINAL PAIN

Narrowing Down and Diagnosis

For the physician, narrowing down the problem of recurrent abdominal pain has been likened to the anguish of the long distance runner (20) and, as is the case with headache, the major effort is to rule out organic pathological disorders. A second concern is to rule out psychogenic pain. The clinician's major tools are a careful history and a thorough physical examination, with some laboratory tests. The history-taking should include the history of the problem and of other illnesses or physical problems, and the family's medical history, with particular attention paid to pain problems. The location, description, and timing of the pain are important. The parents and the child should be interviewed separately to elicit any information that either does not wish to disclose in front of the other. The physical examination should include the measuring of height and weight, and the observation of the child's general appearance. A plot of the weight and height percentile changes can help identify a chronic illness. Masses, enlarged organs, specific locations of tenderness, and hernias should be searched for. A careful perianal examination and rectal examination conclude the physical examination.

Routine laboratory tests for children with recurrent abdominal pain should include complete blood cell count, erythrocyte sedimentation rate, and urinalysis and urine culture. Other laboratory tests should be ordered in response to specific indications, for example, abdominal ultrasound in a young girl with persistent lower quadrant pain. The physician should be aware of the danger of the psychological or physical harm potentially caused by tests that are not necessary. Table 22-3 outlines the general "red flags" that should suggest more thorough follow-up with diagnostic medical investigations (19).

The diagnosis of psychogenic abdominal pain must not be by exclusion but must be based on positive evidence. Psychogenic abdominal pain may occur for any of the reasons mentioned above for psychogenic headache (13).

Narrowing down the problem of psychogenic abdominal pain is accomplished by interview and also by means of a diary (Fig. 22-1) kept by the child and the parents over a period of several weeks. Psychogenic and organic problems may coexist and the finding of one does not exclude the other.

For most children, no organic or psychological cause of recurrent abdominal pain will be found (20). As well, most children with recurrent abdominal pain are psychologically normal (21,22).

Management of recurrent abdominal pain

Pathological abdominal pain should be treated according to its cause. Psychogenic recurrent abdominal pain can be treated by attending to the psychological cause. Children who have recurrent abdominal pain of unknown origin should be entered on a trial of increased fiber in the diet (23). Four weeks of approximately 10 grams of supplementary fiber per day will provide relief in 50% of these children, with few side effects (FIRM EVIDENCE). Fiber can be augmented by increasing the consumption of foods that contain fiber or, more simply, by the addition of fiber biscuits to the diet. If this is not suc-

---

Table 22-3. "Red flags" signaling the need for further investigation in children with stomach pain

History of weight loss and/or reduced appetite
Alteration of function or symptom progression in a specific organ system (e.g., change in bowel habits, polyuria, menstrual problems, vomiting)
Abnormalities of the blood count (e.g., anemia, leukocytosis, elevated erythrocyte sedimentation rate, eosinophilia, altered cellular morphology)
Occult or frank bleeding from any orifice
Abnormal urinalysis and/or culture
Compelling family history of a particular disorder (e.g., ulcer)
Constitutional symptoms of chronic illness (e.g., recurrent fever, ill appearance, growth failure, swollen joints, lack of energy)

From ref. 20 with permission.

PAIN DIARY

Date	What happened before	Pain (How long, where, how severe)	What happened after
Sept 17	Ready to go to school	Doubled over, crying near navel	Rested at home all day
Sept 18	Supper	mild pain	Stopped supper
Sept 23	Dressed for school	Severe pain	stayed home

Figure 22-1. Example of a child's pain diary.

cessful *and* the child is disabled by the pain, referral to a consultant for further organic or psychological investigation is indicated.

COLIC

Narrowing down and diagnosis

Narrowing down the problem of colic requires the exclusion of normal crying and crying that is secondary to another problem. The best way of determining if the baby is crying more, and more often, than normal is to have the parents keep a diary of the amount of time the baby spends crying. Global retrospective reports are likely to be unreliable (22). It is generally accepted that intense crying that lasts for more than 3 hours per day on more than 3 days a week over at least 3 weeks meets the criterion for the excessive crying (6) of colic. Ruling out the pathological causes of excessive crying is best done by history and physical examination. A healthy infant who is gaining at least 150 grams per week in whom all obvious causes of excessive crying have been eliminated can be said to have colic.

Management of colic

Time provides a sure cure for colic since almost all cases of colic spontaneously resolve by the age of 9 months. Two other strategies have been shown to be effective. Instructing parents to try to never let the baby cry and to try and resolve what was bothering the infant, was found to be more effective than advising them to let the child cry (SUGGESTIVE EVIDENCE) (25). Other research provides SUGGESTIVE EVIDENCE (23) that the most important element might be carrying the baby for an additional few hours per day (25). Dicyclomine hydrochloride, with the dose titrated by the parents upward from 1/4 tsp. t.i.d. (1/2 tsp. for babies 8 weeks or older) to a maximum of 1/2 tsp. q.i.d., has been demonstrated to be effective (FIRM EVIDENCE) (27). Concern has been expressed about a possible relationship between dicyclomine and sudden infant death syndrome (NO CLEAR EVIDENCE) and this medication is no longer recommended for children under 3 months old.

A major effort must be made to ensure that the parents realize that colic is a benign, self-limited disorder of unknown physical origin. Parents need reassurance that they are not the cause of the colic, and they need to mobilize their family and friends as resources to help them through this difficult time. Maternal anxiety and overstimulation do not cause colic but might be a response to colic. The book, *Crybabies: Coping with Colic* (28), can be recommended to parents as an excellent resource.

"Gripe water" and phenobarbital-atropine combinations are not recommended; there is NO CLEAR EVIDENCE that they are effective.

CHEST PAIN

Narrowing down and diagnosis

Narrowing down the problem of recurrent chest pain is based on the history and physical examination (7,8,29). Laboratory procedures including chest radiograph and electrocardiogram yield virtually no information unless they are specifically indicated (9), and they have the disadvantage of increasing the anxiety of the child and the parents. The main aim of the primary care physician is to distinguish between treatable disease and benign conditions that require only reassurance and explanation. A physician who understands the benign nature of recurrent chest pain in children will help prevent the child's missing school or otherwise restricting activities (29).

Table 22-4 outlines the key elements in narrowing down the problem of chest pain. Pain that is anginal in nature, accompanied by dyspnea, syncope, or palpitations, should arouse the suspicion of cardiac disease. This is rare in children and the more likely diagnoses are (30) musculoskeletal problems (31% incidence), costochondritis (14%), chest wall syndrome (13%), skeletal trauma (2%), rib-cage anomalies (2%), hyperventilation (20%), breast-related problems (5%), and idiopathic (39%). Other causes of chest pain include chronic or acute respiratory problems, gastrointestinal problems, and psychological problems. Depression (see Chapter 23) may be accompanied by chest pain, and anxiety may trigger hyperventilation (see Chapter 25), but a diagnosis of psychogenic pain must be based on positive evidence.

Management of chest pain

Chest pain due to a specific physical cause should be treated according to standard practice (see Chapters 5, 7, and 9). Benign chest pain should be handled by explaining the condition and reassuring the patient and the parents. Strong directives that the child should return to previous levels of activity are needed to prevent disability. If disability has already occurred and is not responsive to such directives, referral to a consultant is indicated.

Table 22-4. Narrowing down the problem of chest pain

Finding	Narrowing down	Management
Normal physical examination; pain not anginal; no palpitations or dyspnea	Hyperventilation; normal breasts; psychogenic; gastrointestinal	Explanation; reassurance; treat disability
Pain elicited by palpation	Costochondritis; chest wall syndrome; breast problems	Explanation; reassurance; treat disability
Acute pain elicited by respiration	Chest radiograph to diagnose pneumonia, pneumotherax	Treat as indicated
Chronic pain elicited by respiration	Chest radiograph to diagnose allergic, cold, or exercise bronchospasm	Treat as indicated
Angina; syncope; dyspnea; palpitations or fever; cough and friction rub	Myocardial disease; pericarditis; electrocardiogram; chest radiograph	Referral to consultant

LIMB PAIN

Narrowing down and diagnosis

Limb pain can be due to trauma, orthopedic conditions, rheumatic disease, infectious disease, malignancies, benign bony tumors, endocrine disorders, nutritional abnormalities, miscellaneous disorders, syndromes of unknown origin, and psychogenic syndromes (31). Narrowing down the problem is done on the basis of the history, physical examination, and some laboratory tests. Table 22-5 outlines this process. Pain in the knee should always trigger a careful examination of the hip, as the pain may be referred from one joint to the other. Hip pain is discussed in Chapter 8. The three most common limb pain syndromes, which fortunately are benign, are growing pains, patellofemoral pain, and Osgood-Schlatter disease.

Growing pains refer to deep nocturnal pains, usually in the legs, that are severe enough to waken the child from sleep. The pains occur intermittently, are usually bilateral, and are exacerbated by excessive exercise during the day. There are no abnormal physical findings and the pain does not affect daytime activities. Growing pains are not related to the actual physical processes of growing and do not develop into pathologic conditions. The nature of growing pains is unknown.

Patellofemoral pain (often mistakenly called chondromalacia) is diagnosed on the basis of a history of usually anteromedial pain aggravated by stair-climbing, cycling, or prolonged sitting with the knee flexed. There often

Table 22-5. Narrowing down the problem of limb pain

Finding	Narrowing down	Management
Pain in evening or night; pain in thighs, calves, & behind knees; no limp; deep aching, usually bilateral; no local tenderness, redness or swelling; normal, healthy child; usually in 5–12-year-olds	"Growing pains"	Reassurance; analgesics; massage
Recurrent pain in knee(s); worse when walking up stairs or on bike or after prolonged sitting; no local tenderness, redness or swelling; no limp; adolescent girls most frequently affected; normal, healthy child	Patella femoral knee pain	Physiotherapy
Limp	Suspect Legg-Calvé-Perthes disease; radiograph	Referral to consultant
Limp, usually mild pain in knee area; tenderness of tibial tuberosity	Osgood-Schlatter disease; radiograph often not necessary if tibial tuberosity is tender	Rest if severe pain; full activity if tolerated; analgesics before exercise if necessary

is clicking, catching, or giving way; there may be locking. Persistent effusion is not characteristic, and there are no systemic findings or atrophy. The adolescent female athlete is probably the most frequent sufferer. It is hypothesized that the problem stems from malalignment and subsequent abnormalities of patellar tracking. True chondromalacia of the patella does occur but is an infrequent cause of patellofemoral pain.

Osgood-Schlatter disease (see Chapter 8 as well) is marked by pain, swelling, and tenderness in the tibial tuberosity. There is often a limp. Pressure on the tibial tuberosity that produces the pain is virtually diagnostic. The radiograph will usually show an abnormal tibial tuberosity but is unnecessary in the typical case.

Management of limb pain

Growing pains are managed by reassurance, heat, massage, and acetylsalicylic acid or acetaminophen.

There is NO CLEAR EVIDENCE that strengthening of the quadriceps or surgical release benefits patients with patellofemoral pain. However, conservative treatment, including strengthening of the quadriceps and avoidance of knee flexion, is preferable to more invasive surgical procedures.

Osgood-Schlatter disease is treated by having the patient avoid activities that cause pain or take analgesics prior to exercise. There is NO CLEAR EVIDENCE that children who continue activity in the face of pain do themselves any harm.

CHRONIC PAIN SYNDROME

Narrowing down

The vast majority of children with long-term pain continue to function well socially and academically. Recent investigations in both pediatric migraine (32) and in recurrent abdominal pain (21,22) have demonstrated that, as a group, children with chronic benign pain are psychologically similar to other children.

There is, however, a small subset of children who do not fare as well. These children miss school, withdraw from social activities, become preoccupied with their pain, and begin early to launch their careers as pain patients. The families of these children are frequently as involved in the process as are the children. "Doctor shopping" and, at times, unnecessary treatments are undertaken in vain searches for a cure for the pain (33).

Such children have been described as having psychogenic pain (34), but it may be more accurate to refer to them as chronic pain patients. Chronic pain patients may have pain in any area, and not infrequently the pain occurs in multiple or changing sites. The pain may be of organic or psychogenic etiology, but the essential factor is that any physical findings are not sufficient to explain the incapacity. The patients cope poorly with the pain and require assistance to lessen the disruption that the pain causes in their lives.

Management of chronic pain syndrome

The crucial element in the management of the care of a child with chronic pain syndrome is rapid intervention to prevent the development of major secondary problems due to family disruption and absence from school. In most cases, treatment is carried out by a consultant.

REFERENCES

1. King, H.A. Back pain in children. *Pediatr. Clin. North Am.* 31:1083–1095, 1984.
2. Bille, B. Migraine in schoolchildren. *Acta Pediatr. Scand.* 51 (suppl. 136):1–151, 1962.
3. Sillanpaa, M. Changes in the prevalence of migraine and other headache during the first seven school years. *Headache* 23:15–19, 1983.

4. Oster, J. Recurrent abdominal pain, headache and limb pain in children and adolescents. *Pediatrics* 50:429–436, 1972.

5. Apley, J., Hale, B. Children with recurrent abdominal pains: A field survey of 1000 school children. *Arch. Dis. Child.* 33:165–170, 1958.

6. Wessel, M.A., Cobb, J.C., Jackson, E.B., Harris, G.S., Detwiler, A.C. Paroxysmal fussing in infancy, sometimes called colic. *Pediatrics* 14:421–434, 1954.

7. Coleman, W.L. Recurrent chest pain in children. *Pediatr. Clin. North Am.* 31:1007–1026, 1984.

8. Brenner, J.I., Engel, R.E., Berman, M.A. Cardiologic perspectives of chest pain in childhood: A referral problem? To whom? *Pediatr. Clin. North Am.* 31:1241–1258, 1984.

9. Naish, J.M., Apley, J. "Growing pains." A clinical study of non-arthritic limb pains in children. *Arch. Dis. Child.* 26:134–140, 1951.

10. McGrath, P.J. Migraine headaches in children and adolescents. In *Advances in Behavioral Medicine for Children and Adolescents*, Firestone, P., McGrath, P.J. Feldman, W., eds. Hillsdale, N.J.: Lawrence Erlbaum Associates, 1983.

11. Gascon, G.G. Chronic and recurrent headache in children and adolescents. *Pediatr. Clin. North Am.* 31:1027–1051, 1984.

12. Barlow, C.F. Headaches and migraine in childhood. *Clin. in Dev. Med.* 91 London: Spastics International Medical Publications, 1984.

13. McGrath, P.J. Psychological aspects of recurrent abdominal pain. *Canadian Family Physician* 29:1655–1659, 1983.

14. Ludvigsson, J. Propranolol used in prophylaxis of migraine in children. *Acta Neurol. Scand.* 50:109–115, 1974.

15. Forsythe, W.I., Gillies, D., Sills, M.A. Propranolol (Inderal) in the treatment of childhood migraine. *Dev. Med. Child Neurol.* 26:737–741, 1984.

16. Couch, J.R., Hassanein, R.S. Amitriptyline in migraine prophylaxis. *Arch. Neurol.* 36:695–699, 1979.

17. Drugs for migraine. *Med. Lett. Drugs Ther.* 26:95–96, 1984.

18. Richter, I., McGrath, P.J., Humphreys, P., Goodman, J.T., Firestone, P., Keene, D. Cognitive and relaxation treatment of paediatric migraine. *Pain* 25:195–203, 1986.

19. Andrasik, F., Blake, D.D., McCarran, M.S. A biobehavioral analysis of pediatric headache. In *Child Health Behavior: A Behavioral Pediatrics Perspective.* Krasnegor, N.A., Cataldo, M.F., Arasteh, J.D. eds. New York: Wiley 394–434, 1986.

20. Levine, M., Rappaport, L.A. Recurrent abdominal pain in school children: The loneliness of the long distance physician. *Pediatr. Clin. North Am.* 31:969–991, 1984.

21. McGrath, P.J., Goodman, J.T., Firestone, P., Shipman, R., Peters, S. Recurrent abdominal pain: A psychogenic disorder? *Arch. Dis. Child.* 58:888–890, 1983.

22. Raymer, D., Weininger, O., Hamilton, J.R. Psychological problems in children with abdominal pain. *Lancet* 1:439–440, 1984.

23. Barr, R.G., Feuerstein, M. Recurrent abdominal pain syndrome: How appropriate are our basic clinical assumptions? In *Pediatric and Adolescent Behavioral Medicine: Issues in Treatment*, McGrath, P., Firestone, P., eds. New York: Springer, 1983.

24. Feldman, W., McGrath, P.J., Hodgson, C., Ritter, H., Shipman, R.T. The use of dietary fiber in the management of simple childhood idiopathic recurrent abdominal pain: Results in a prospective double blind randomized controlled trial. *Am. J. Dis. Child.* 139:1216–1218, 1985.

25. Taubman, B. Clinical trial of the treatment of colic by modification of parent-infant interaction. *Pediatrics* 74:998–1003, 1984.

26. Hunziker, U.A., Barr, R.G. Increased carrying reduces infant crying: A randomized controlled trial. *Pediatrics*, 77:641–648, 1985.
27. Weissbluth, M., Christoffel, K.K., Davis, A.T. Treatment of infantile colic with dicyclomine hydrochloride. *J. Pediatr.* 104:951–955, 1984.
28. Weissbluth, M. *Crybabies: Coping with Colic*. New York: Arbor House, 1984.
29. Selbst, S.M. Chest pain in children. *Pediatrics* 75:1068–1070, 1985.
30. Pantell, R.H., Goodman, B.W. Adolescent chest pain: A prospective study. *Pediatrics* 71:881–887, 1983.
31. Bowyer, S.L., Hollister, R. Limb pain in childhood. *Pediatr. Clin. North Am.* 31:1053–1081, 1984.
32. Cunningham, S.J., McGrath, P.J., Ferguson, R.B., et al. Personality and behavioral characteristics in paediatric migraine. *Headache* 27:16–20, 1987.
33. McGrath, P.J., Dunn-Geier, J., Cunningham, S.J., Brunette, R., D'Astous, J., Humphreys, P., Latter, J., Keene, D. Psychological guidelines for helping children cope with chronic benign intractable pain. *Clin. J. Pain* 1:229–233, 1985.
34. Green, M. Sources of pain. In *Developmental-Behavioral Pediatrics*, Levine, M.D., Carey, W.B., Crocker, A.C., Gross, R.T., eds. Philadelphia: W.B. Saunders, 1983, pp. 512–518.

23

ANXIETY AND DEPRESSION

Anxiety and depression are internalizing problems, in contrast to the externalizing problems dealt with in Chapter 20. Anxiety and depression are unpleasant thoughts or feelings that may be accompanied by behavioral manifestations.

Anxiety ranges from normal reactions, such as separation anxiety in the 2-year-old, to the serious pathological reactions of the schizophrenic child. There is controversy as to whether the depression seen in adults exists as a syndrome in children, but there is little doubt that some children do have depressive thoughts and feelings such as pessimism, moodiness, wanting to die, and unhappiness. They may exhibit depressive behaviors such as crying, sleep disturbance, eating problems, and motor retardation.

PREVALENCE

Childhood fears or anxieties that interfere with activities occur in various forms in more than one-third of children aged 2 to 14 years (1). Almost all children at one time or another have some specific fears. Most childhood fears should be regarded as part of normal development or a normal variant of personality or temperament (2); they include stranger anxiety at about 6 months and separation anxiety between 12 and 15 months, the fear of small animals that occurs in children not exposed to pets, and the common fear of ghosts or monsters. The prevalence of childhood depression has been estimated to range from 0.02 to 12% (3).

Although the cognitive and behavioral aspects of both anxiety and depression frequently coincide, it is not unusual for children, especially older children, to report anxiety or depression and still behave in a nonfearful or nondepressed way or vice versa. The key issue in determining whether or not the anxiety or depression should be treated is the degree to which the problem interferes with the life of the child or the family.

207

The long-term prognosis, in terms of normal functioning as adults, for children who have anxiety, fear, or depression is substantially better than that for children exhibiting antisocial or acting-out behavior (4). However, it is also clear that children who do not acquire appropriate social skills (because of anxiety or avoidance, for example) are at risk of developing psychological problems later (5). Social isolation, or being a loner, in and of itself has not clearly been shown to be predictive of maladjustment (6).

ANXIETY

Narrowing down

At least five types of anxiety or withdrawal are observed in children: separation anxiety, generalized anxiety, specific phobias, social anxiety, and anxiety associated with psychosis (Table 23-1).

Narrowing down the problem of anxiety is done on the basis of reports from the child, the teacher, and the family. Detailed descriptions of the occurrences of the problem and their context should be solicited. A very important component of the narrowing down process is determining how much of a problem the anxiety or withdrawal is and for whom it is a problem. Treatment is not indicated unless the anxiety interferes with the child's own life or the family's life.

Parents will frequently feel more at ease discussing their concerns and speculations when the child is not present. Children will sometimes be more candid when the parents are absent and they have assurances of confidentiality. Thus separate interviews for the parents and the child are recommended.

The child's teacher can be telephoned or can be asked to fill out a standard behavior scale, such as the Child Behavior Checklist (7).

Separation anxiety Separation anxiety is the normal response of an infant or young child to separation from his or her primary caretaker. Separation anxiety normally beings at about 12 to 15 months and, depending on the child's experience and temperament, will decline over the second to fourth years of life. Separation anxiety is usually manifested by fussing and crying when the mother leaves the child's presence. The child can be calmed within a few minutes by the babysitter's or other caretaker's judicious distraction and comforting. Extreme or abnormal separation anxiety occurs when the child maintains the fear of separation well past the second year and cannot be distracted or comforted.

Separation anxiety is frequently manifested when the child first attends a day-care center or school. This anxiety often recurs following a period spent at home during vacation or illness and is known as school phobia. Not all children who refuse to go to school have a school phobia. Some are truants who have discovered more rewarding things to do than to go to school. Others have specific realistic fears of being beaten up or teased. Often children who

Table 23-1. Anxiety problems in children

Type of anxiety	Narrowing down	Management
Separation anxiety	Distress at separation from caregiver	
Normal	Begins 12–15 months; occurs in new situations, e.g. day care; resolves with warm, firm handling	Parental reassurance
Extreme (including Type 1 school phobia)	Result of deception or inadvertent reinforcement of anxiety behavior; recent onset; otherwise OK; child younger than 10 years	Repeated separation; reinforcement of correct behavior; distraction
Complex, learned (including Type 2 school phobia)	Result of family disorganization or dysfunction; chronic problems; child older than 10 years	Referral to consultant
Generalized anxiety	Anxiety provoked by almost anything or nothing at all	
Temperamental	Early onset; pervasive	Encourage to face anxiety; relief for parent
Stress-induced	Response to personal or family stress	Resolve stress
Depressive accompaniment	Evidence that depression is primary	Treat depression
Specific phobias		
Developmental	Stranger anxiety at six months of age	Reassurance
Minor	Fears do not interfere with activities	No treatment
Major	Irrational fears interfere with child's or family's life	Exposure treatment; adjunctive pharmocotherapy
Pseudophobia	Skill deficits cause anxiety	Teach skill
Social anxiety	Anxiety about people	
Normal shyness	Child is slow to warm up, reticent; has some social relationships	Acceptance of normal variation; encouragement
Severe shyness	Shyness limits most social encounters and inhibits activites in other areas such as school and sports	Encouragement and support to find areas of successful social interaction; referral to consultant
Pathological	Social interaction totally limited; bizarre behavior	Referral to consultant

are absent from school because of school phobia complain of headaches or stomach aches that coincide with the parents' demand that they go to school and wane when the demand is retracted. These somatic complaints are often genuine results of anxiety, but they may be used as an avoidance tactic (see Chapter 22).

Kennedy (8) delineated two types of school phobia. Type 1, or simple school phobia, is characterized by sudden onset in a young child, usually following a legitimate absence from school because of illness or vacation. In such cases, the family is psychologically normal and the parents cooperate with each other in child care. Type 2, complex school phobia, occurs in older children whose family relationships are disturbed and who have a chronic history of gradually increasing absences from school.

Generalized anxiety Generalized anxiety refers to a strong fear of a wide variety of situations. The child may react with protestations and distress to being dressed in a different set of clothes, to being fed a new food, or to being put to bed by a new person. If the pattern is long-standing, it is most likely the result of temperament (the constitutional and persevering element of personality [2,9]). If the problem is of recent origin, a specific stress may have triggered a widespread anxiety reaction.

Specific phobia A specific phobia is a strong fear of a specific stimulus. Some of the more common phobias are fear of animals, most often dogs, mice or snakes; fear of the dark; and fear of public speaking. Often these fears can be traced to a specific traumatic situation, but this is not always the case nor is it necessary to know the cause for the problem to be addressed.

Social anxiety Social anxiety can range from the normal, expected stranger anxiety at around 6 months of age to severe pathology in the totally withdrawn autistic or schizophrenic child. There is a great deal of normal variation in the amount and type of social interaction in which people choose to engage. Normal shyness (defined as shyness that does not interfere with a child's family, academic, or social functioning) frequently runs in families and is not pathological (10).

Children who are unhappy about their reticence or who avoid attending family, academic, and social functions can be considered abnormally shy. Social anxiety about the opposite sex is common in adolescents and, unless accompanied by a more pervasive withdrawal, should not be considered problematic.

Anxiety secondary to psychosis Widespread anxiety or severe specific anxiety may occur in autism or childhood schizophrenia. Children with these conditions also have pervasive and severe thought, language, and personality disturbances and should be referred to a consultant.

Anxiety, depression and behavior disorders Differentiating between anxiety, depression, and behavior disorders is often difficult and sometimes impossible. Severe anxiety may lead to depressed mood, and depressed mood may lead to the avoidance of many situations. Depression may, at times, be associated with acting-out behavior, and behavior problems may be accompanied by low mood. Judging the primacy of depression, anxiety, or behavior problems is often a matter of which of the three is more pervasive.

Management of anxiety

Anxiety is most frequently managed by psychological means but, on occasion, pharmacological or a combination of psychological and pharmacological strategies is more effective.

Separation anxiety Parental concern about separation anxiety in infants and young children can be dealt with by the primary care physician's reassuring them that normal separation anxiety is to be expected and that a child's crying should not cause them to feel guilty. Parents should be advised not to avoid leaving the child with another caregiver. Repeated "giving in" to a child who cries when his or her parents leave may only teach the child that crying can control the parents' behavior. Parents should be advised *never* to deceive a child in order to avoid a show of separation anxiety. If a child is deceived once about the parents' leaving, the child will never know when the parents will leave in the future and will not trust any reassurances they give.

A child who develops extreme separation anxiety, either because of having been reinforced in the behavior by the parents or because he or she was deceived, may need a period of reeducation in which there is ample opportunity to learn both that crying will not prevent the parents from leaving and that the parents will return. Parents may need considerable reassurance that their child will not be harmed by the separation. It is also crucial to ensure that one of the parents is not encouraging separation anxiety by separating tentatively and returning when the child cries.

The following are the basic steps that parents should follow in dealing with separation anxiety:

1. Inform the child you are leaving. Depending on his or her age, this may mean telling the child where you are going and when you will return or simply saying "bye-bye."
2. Leave and do not be swayed by protests.
3. The child should be comforted, reassured, and then quickly distracted into some pleasant activity by the adult who remains with the child.
4. Extra attention should be given by the parents to the child at other times.

There is NO CLEAR EVIDENCE of the validity of this approach. Adjunctive short-term pharmacological treatment may help smooth the reeducation process (NO CLEAR EVIDENCE). However, pharmacotherapy can *never* substitute for appropriate behavioral guidance and should *never* be used as the sole treatment (11). Diphenhydramine (5 mg/kg/24 hours in three doses) is the safest and most effective treatment, with hydroxyzine (2 mg/kg/24 hours in three doses) as a second choice (11).

Kennedy's treatment approach to simple school phobia can be implemented by the primary care physician and involves the following elements:

1. Intervention begun as soon after the problem is noticed as possible. Early intervention will prevent secondary problems arising from the child's missing work at school, from enjoying staying at home, from social isolation, or from embarrassment.
2. A deemphasis of somatic complaints and an insistence that the child persist at school in spite of discomfort.
3. Resolution of realistic aspects of the school avoidance, such as protection from bullies.
4. Decisive insistence on going to school, even if physical force is required.
5. Close liaison with the parents to ensure that they take a nonemotional but firm approach and make the child go to school.
6. Parents, teachers, and the physician providing positive feedback to the child for school attendance.
7. Follow-up to ensure consolidation of the child's gains in his or her battle against fear.

Kennedy (8) reported that 100% of 50 children with Type 1, or simple, school phobia were successfully returned to and kept in school using the above program (SUGGESTIVE EVIDENCE). A gradual approach in which the return to full-time school attendance is done in small steps is an alternative. A gradual approach may be less stressful to the child and family but it may allow for the development of secondary problems such as falling behind in studies. A child who misses school because of complex school phobia (chronic history of gradually increasing school avoidance combined with disturbed family relationships) will probably require extensive therapy and should be referred to a consultant.

Pharmacological treatment, using imipramine (1 to 3 mg/kg/24 hours) is also effective when used in conjunction with concerted efforts to return the child to school (FIRM EVIDENCE) (11). HOWEVER, THERE IS A HIGH POTENTIAL FOR TRICYCLIC ANTIDEPRESSANT POISONING RESULTING FROM DELIBERATE OR ACCIDENTAL INGESTION. CARE MUST BE TAKEN IN PRESCRIBING TRICYCLICS TO CHILDREN AT RISK FOR SUICIDE, AND CAUTIONS MUST BE GIVEN THE FAMILIES OF YOUNG CHILDREN ABOUT SAFE HOME STORAGE OF SUCH DRUGS.

Generalized anxiety A child who cannot adapt to new situations and instead withdraws is best handled with warm but firm direction. The child should be encouraged to engage in the behaviors he or she fears and discouraged from avoiding new situations. Parents should be cautioned not to ridicule the child, as this is likely to cause problems with self-esteem. Perhaps most important for the parents is reassurance that an avoidant and nonadaptive temperament in a child is a normal biological variant and is not due to parental deficiencies (2,9). Pharmacological treatment is not recommended for normal or temperamental anxiety.

Specific phobias The basic principle of management in specific anxiety is to expose the child to the feared stimulus without there being a way for him or her to escape or avoid the situation (FIRM EVIDENCE) (12). To enhance the probability of successful exposure and to reduce any negative side effects, it is usually best to gradually expose the child to the stimulus in combination with positive reinforcement for progressive adaptation to whatever is feared. For example, a child who is very afraid of water because he or she accidentally aspirated water while swimming could be gradually reintroduced to the water by at first being encouraged to play at the edge of the pool and then, little by little—with praise and attention for progress—induced to play in deeper water. Eventually, the child will be quite comfortable with full participation in the water. Fear of the doctor or dentist because of an adverse experience can be treated in the same manner, by progressive adaptation. The initial appointments should not include an examination and treatment; they should merely introduce the child to the physician or dentist in an encouraging environment. Later, examinations and treatment can be undertaken.

As a general rule, in cases of moderate or severe anxiety or fear, forced, immediate exposure to the maximally feared event (flooding) is *not* encouraged. Although flooding is effective treatment (FIRM EVIDENCE) (12) in the hands of experienced therapists treating adults' phobias, it can be extremely painful for the child and for the parents. As well, the child may escape because he or she becomes so upset that the parents feel the child must be allowed to escape. In some cases, the child may escape flooding by becoming hysterical or by fainting.

A distinction should be made between situations that are avoided because of fear and those that are avoided because the child accurately perceives his or her lack of the skills needed to participate successfully in the activity. Exposure will assist in overcoming anxiety but will not correct a problem due to a lack of knowledge of skill. For example, a child who is afraid of speaking up in class because he or she does not know the answer is not suffering from anxiety but from a lack of knowledge. Similarly, many other phobias may involve a knowledge or skill component. A fear of deep water may partially be alleviated by learning how to swim. When the knowledge of a skill is a component of anxiety, a gradual approach, in which the skill is taught as well as exposure provided, is appropriate.

Adjunctive pharmacotherapy (NO CLEAR EVIDENCE) can also be used on a temporary basis. Diphenhydramine or hydroxyzine in the dosages previously mentioned are recommended for younger children, and thioridazine (1 mg/kg/24 hours in three doses) is recommended for older children and adolescents (11).

Social anxiety   Normal shyness should be accepted with positive and gentle encouragement that the child do as much as he or she can. It is important for parents to realize that shyness is a normal behavioral variant that is a part of the child's inborn personality. Parents should pay attention to the child's social initiation and be careful not to criticize the behavior of children who are naturally shy. Children who are shy are probably in even greater need of the warmth, recognition, and predictability of circumstance that all children need. If the child is a regular patient of the physician and knows the physician, it may be possible for the physician to discuss directly with the child the factors that contribute to the shyness and suggest ways to help the child face more situations.

Severe shyness that interferes with a child's academic, family, or social life deserves more deliberate intervention. Depending on the exact nature and extent of the shyness, the parents can be encouraged to develop opportunities for the child such as participating in small play groups, having individual friends to the home, or enrolling in an activity the child enjoys. In some cases, the shy child will benefit from being given the chance to talk to the physician about the problem. However, most children will overcome shyness only in a social situation. Pharmacotherapy is not recommended. Referral to a mental health consultant familiar with social problems should be considered.

Pathological social anxiety is marked by extreme avoidance of virtually all social interaction. Referral to a mental health consultant is indicated, as such symptoms may be indicative of mental illness. In any event, prolonged intensive treatment will be required.

DEPRESSION

Five types of depression occur in children (Table 23-2). The first is very extreme mood swings, which are normal for some children and adolescents. Despair that seems to arise for no substantial reason may be replaced 10 hours later by elation, also arising for no apparent reason. The second is the depressed mood that follows some setback or loss. The moving away of a friend or failing a test may result in depressed mood for several days or even weeks. The third is the more long-term depressive mood, which often is very pervasive and arises for no apparent reason.

The last two types are "normal" suicidal thoughts and dangerous suicidal thoughts. No matter what the type of depressed behavior, it is important to

Table 23-2. Depressive problems in children

Type of problem	Narrowing down	Management
Normal mood swings	Changes in mood; may be extreme, but last only a few hours or 1-2 days	Reassurance
Reaction to loss or failure	Identifiable crisis; may last for months if crisis is severe	Reassurance, support
Chronic depression	Long-lasting, inconsolable, no good reason for mood	Referral
Suicidal thoughts (normal)	Occasional; no definite plans or gestures	Reassurance, follow up
Suicidal thoughts (dangerous)	Constant, or accompanied by definite plans or gestures	Referral

ask the parent and the child about thoughts or plans of suicide. Children will readily accept and will usually answer such questions as, "Have you ever thought of harming yourself?" "Normal" suicidal thoughts may occur with mood swings and will not be accompanied by well-developed plans or actual suicide attempts. Dangerous suicidal thoughts are accompanied by specific plans and/or suicidal gestures.

Depression in children has been measured by the self-report scales developed by Birelson (13) and Kovacs (14), the interview schedule developed by Poznanski (15), and the parental report scale of Wirt et al. (16), but none of these have gained widespread acceptance in clinical practice.

Management of depression

Normal depressive moods No treatment, other than reassurance that such moods are normal, is appropriate for normal depressive moods unless there has been persistent thinking about and planning of suicide.

Depression due to loss Common sense supports the notion that a kind listener who is supportive and understanding is probably the best treatment for depression due to loss (NO CLEAR EVIDENCE).

Long-term depressive mood The use of imipramine (1 to 3 mg/kg/24 hours, once daily at bedtime) is supported by some SUGGESTIVE EVIDENCE (17,18) of its efficacy in childhood depression of all types. Amitryptyline is also useful at the same dosage (SUGGESTIVE EVIDENCE) (19).

Talk of suicide Talk of suicide should never be ignored or dismissed but should always be assessed thoroughly to determine the extent of the motivation. Suicidal thoughts that come and go but are not accompanied by specific plans and have not been acted on are very common and do require exploration to determine what is triggering them. Specific plans of suicide and any attempts must be seen as *dangerous* and should immediately be assessed by a specialist.

A child with severe depression for no discernible reason, in which there are mood and vegetative signs lasting for more than 2 to 3 weeks and/or definite suicidal plans or gestures, should be referred to a consultant.

REFERENCES

1. Macfarlane, J.W., Allen, L., Honzick, M. *A Developmental Study of the Behavior Problems of Normal Children*. Berkeley: University of California Press, 1954.
2. Thomas, A., Chess, S., Birch, H.G. *Temperament and Behavior Disorders in Children*. London: University of London Press, 1968.
3. Petti, T.A. Active treatment of childhood depression. In *Depression: Behavioral and Directive Strategies*, Clarkin, J.F., Glazer, H.I., eds. New York: Garland, 1981.
4. Robins, L.N. *Deviant Children Grow Up*. Baltimore: Williams and Wilkins, 1966.
5. Cartledge, C., Milburn, J.F. *Teaching Social Skills to Children*. New York: Pergamon, 1980.
6. French, D.C., Tyne, T.F. The identification and treatment of children with peer-relationship difficulties. In *Social Skills Training: A Practical Handbook for Assessment and Treatment*, Curran, J.P., Monti, P.M., eds. New York: Guilford, 1982, pp. 280–308.
7. Achenbach, T.M., Edelbrock, C.S. The child behavior profile: II Boys aged 12–16 and girls 6–11 and 12–16. *J. Consulting and Clinical Psychology* 47:223–233, 1979.
8. Kennedy, W.A. School phobia: Rapid treatment of fifty cases. *J. Abnorm. Psychol.* 70:285–289, 1965.
9. Chess, S., Thomas, A. Dynamics of individual behavioral development. In *Developmental-Behavioral Pediatrics*, Levine, M.D., Carey, W.B., Crocker, A.C., Gross, R.T., eds. Philadelphia: W.B. Saunders, 1983, pp. 158–175.
10. Zimbardo, P. *Shyness: What It Is: What To Do About It*. Reading, Mass.: Addison-Wesley, 1977.
11. White, J.H. Pharmacology in childhood: Current status and future prospectives. *Psychiatr. Clin. North Am.* 3:443–453, 1980.
12. Marshall, W.L., Gauthier, J., Gordon, A. The current status of flooding therapy. In *Progress in Behavior Modification*, vol. 7, Hersen, M., Eisler, R.M., Miller, P.M., eds. New York: Academic Press, 1979, pp. 205–275.
13. Birelson, P. The validity of depressive disorders in childhood and the development of a self rating scale: A research report. *J. Child Psychol. Psychiatry* 22:73–88, 1981.
14. Kovacs, M. Rating scales to assess depression in school aged children. *Acta Paedopsychiatr.* 46:305–315, 1981.
15. Poznanski, E.O., Cook, S.C., Carrol, B.J. A depression rating scale for children. *Pediatrics* 64:442–450, 1979.
16. Wirt, R.D., Lachar, D., Klinedinst, J.K., Seat, P.D. *Multidimensional Description of*

Child Personality: A Manual for the Personality Inventory for Children. Los Angeles: Western Psychological Services, 1977.

17. Gittleman-Klein, R., Klein, D.F. School phobia: Diagnostic considerations in the light of imipramine effects. *J. Nerv. Ment. Dis.* 150:199–215, 1973.

18. Petti, T.A. Imipramine in the treatment of depressed children. In *Childhood Depression*, Cantwell, D.P., Carlson, G., eds. New York: Spectrum, 1980.

19. Aylward, G.P. Understanding and treatment of childhood depression. *J. Pediatr.* 107:1–9, 1985.

24

CHILDHOOD INJURIES

Traditionally called accidents, injuries in children demonstrate epidemiological patterns, often are preventable, and constitute the single largest cause of death in children, accounting for more than four times as many deaths as any other single cause. In the United States, 22,000 children under 19 years of age die each year from injuries. For every death, 1,270 children are treated in a medical facility for injuries and 44 are admitted to a hospital for treatment (1).

This chapter highlights the common causes of accidental injuries in children in four age groups: birth to 1 year, 1 to 4 years, 5 to 14 years, and 15 to 19 years. The frequencies and common causes of death differ considerably among the four age groups, but prevention in all four groups is best achieved by altering the environmental settings where injuries are likely to happen. The discussion of each cause is followed by the presentation of the best-known strategy for preventing the injury, with an assessment of the known efficacy of the intervention.

BIRTH TO 1 YEAR

Of the total of 21,962 injury-related deaths in the United States in 1980, 1,166, or 5.9%, occurred in children under age 1 (Table 24-1).

Choking/suffocation

Approximately 10% of all injury-related deaths result from choking on inhaled foreign bodies; 30% of injury-related deaths in infants are from choking. Objects that choke infants include coins, plants, safety pins, uninflated balloons, baby aspirin, pull-tabs on beverage cans, eggshells, and baby powder (2). The larynx is the most likely anatomic site for obstruction in this age group. The preferred lifesaving maneuver for a choking infant remains controversial. Three maneuvers have been advocated, but only when obstruction of the airway is complete.

Table 24-1. Deaths from injuries in children from birth to 1 year

Cause	Percent of deaths	Prevention strategy	Quality of evidence
Choking/suffocation	38	Back blow–chest thrust maneuver	No clear evidence
Motor vehicle accident	19	Counseling	Suggestive evidence
		Seat-belt law	Firm evidence
Burns	15	Education	No clear evidence
Drowning	8	Parental education	No clear evidence
Falls	4	Parental counseling	Suggestive evidence
Poisoning	2	Parental counseling	No clear evidence
Other	14		

Back blow and chest thrust   The infant should be held at a 60° angle, with the head down and the anterior of the body on the rescuer's upper leg. A blow to dislodge the foreign body should be delivered with the heel of the hand to the spine above the shoulder blades. After four back blows, the infant should be turned over and two fingers placed on the sternum to deliver four rapid chest thrusts, similar to the method used for external cardiac message. If the child fails to breathe after this sequence, the mouth should be cleared of foreign material and, after four mouth-to-mouth lung inflations, the sequence of back blows and chest thrusts should be repeated. This maneuver is the one currently recommended by several major health and professional organizations (3). However, there is NO CLEAR EVIDENCE that it is more effective than those described below.

Abdominal thrust   The abdominal thrust, or Heimlich maneuver, is administered with the infant on his or her back in the head-down position. The fist is thrust into the abdomen just below the xiphoid process using four rapid increases in pressure. There is NO CLEAR EVIDENCE of this maneuver's efficacy (4). The maneuver produces five times less pressure in the larynx than does a normal cough.

A theoretically superior maneuver suggested by Day that involves downward blows to the shoulders remains unassessed (5).

Prevention of choking   The two approaches to the prevention of choking are (a) instructing the parents about the hazards of foreign body aspiration, and making them familiar with the common objects that cause obstruction and with the need to make sure that an infant's food is pureed or cut into small pieces; and (b), instructing the parents about how to perform the back blow–

chest thrust maneuver. Attempts to demonstrate the impact of community-wide "heart saver baby" programs have produced NO CLEAR EVIDENCE that they reduce mortality (6). Common sense suggests that increased awareness among parents of how to prevent choking and what to do in the event of choking may reduce the death toll.

Motor vehicle injuries

Nineteen percent of deaths of infants under 1 year of age occur in motor vehicles. The incidence peaks at the age of 2 months (7). An adult holding a 10-pound baby in a collision at 30 miles per hour would need the strength required to lift 300 pounds to hold onto the baby. Clearly, infants in motor vehicles should wear proper restraints, beginning the day the newborn leaves the hospital.

Several studies of extensive physician counseling have found NO CLEAR EVIDENCE of significant improvements in parents' compliance with instructions to use restraints (8). However, legislation requiring child restraints has resulted in FIRM EVIDENCE of improvement in compliance (9). In one study, in which physicians' counseling began at birth, there was SUGGESTIVE EVIDENCE of improved use of restraints for up to 15 months (10). Physicians can advocate for supportive legislation as well as counsel their patients regarding the use of restraints for infants in motor vehicles.

Burns

Fifteen percent of injury-related deaths involve burns. Infants are at greatest risk for burns in house fires, over half of which are caused by careless cigarette smoking. Scalds from tap water, burns from heating or cooking stoves, and the ignition of flammable clothing constitute risks for infants.

Physicians should counsel parents against use of cotton clothing or loose nightgowns because they are flammable and burn rapidly. Purchase of flame-retardant clothing should also be advised. Advocacy of smoke detector use and informing parents of the risk of scalds or burns are unproven preventive strategies. Immediate application of cold water to the burn area will reduce extension of the burn.

Drowning

Drowning accounts for 6% of deaths in this age group, and drowning in the bath tub accounts for most of this mortality. In one survey, children in large families were at highest risk, with most incidents occurring when an older sibling was supervising the bath (11).

When a child is discovered drowning, immediate cardiopulmonary resuscitation (CPR) should be implemented. If all parents were trained in CPR ("heart saver baby") the loss of life might be lessened, but there is NO CLEAR EVIDENCE to support this statement. Other than general parental education, no specific prevention programs have been assessed for the prevention of drowning.

Falls

Falls account for 4% of injuries to infants. Death and serious injury almost always result from head injuries. The most common falls are from cribs or changing tables, down stairs, or out windows.

Legislation of building codes requiring proper handrail protection and gates or doors on stairwells, as well as window guards, would reduce stair and window falls. One house inspection campaign found 30% of homes inspected deficient according to existing building codes (12).

There is SUGGESTIVE EVIDENCE that physicians' counseling parents about stair gates, window guards, safe cribs, elimination of the changing table (parents should use the floor), and adjustment of the level of the crib mattress can reduce falls (13).

Poisoning

Poisoning remains a relatively common problem. About 30% of all poisonings in children occur in those less than 1 year old. Thirty-seven percent of poisonings involve medicine, 37% household cleaning agents, and 25% ingestion of plants (14).

The introduction of safety caps in the 1970s significantly reduced the incidence of poisonings in children. There is SUGGESTIVE EVIDENCE that one-to-one physician-patient counseling about the risk of poisoning does not produce a significant decrease in home poisonings (15). Unfortunately, two large-scale projects in California and Massachusetts produced SUGGESTIVE EVIDENCE that community education resulted in no significant reduction in poisonings (16). Although there is NO CLEAR EVIDENCE to support the practice, most experts encourage parents to keep syrup of ipecac in the home. Parents should seek advice from a poison control center or from their physician about how to use the syrup (17). Use of gastric lavage is contraindicated for corrosives. Lavage is controversial for petroleum-based substances while emesis is contraindicated for them.

Battering

Twenty-five percent of all fractures in children under 3 years of age have been attributed to child battering; 66% of all cases of battering occur in children under 3 years of age and one-third in children under 6 months of age (Fig. 24-1) (1). Skeletal injuries from child battering have specific characteristics due to the mechanism of the injury, which is either a pull, a twist or shearing force, or a direct blow. Direct blows to the ribcage or the head result in fractures in these areas that are very rarely caused by any other mechanism. Battered children are often poorly nourished and somewhat underweight, and there may be poor bone formation. Their general condition results in injuries that are almost always in the metaphysis of the bone and rarely affect the growth plates at the joints. Child battering injuries are also characterized by the finding on skeletal radiographs of a number of fractures in various stages of healing. The physician should suspect battering in any child under age 3 who has a single fracture and a vague history of injury; a skeletal radiographic survey should be obtained to rule out the presence of other fractures.

Fractures usually occur when the arms are held back as the child is shaken. These forces, combined with the child's squirming, produce both longitudinal traction and a shearing action that lead to metaphyseal fractures of the humerus, which may be spiral and are often midshaft. Figure 24-1 shows the frequency and location of fractures from a survey of 74 children who were battered; each child has an average of 3.6 fractures. The most common fracture found was of the ribs, caused by a direct blow to the ribcage. A fractured sternum in a child almost never occurs unless there is a direct blow to the chest. Rib fractures are characteristically posterolateral, since a direct blow to the anterior or posterior ribcage causes flaring and fracture in the midaxillary line. Further guidelines for the detection of child abuse and of families at risk for child abuse are included in Chapter 14.

1 TO 4 YEARS

Of the 21,962 injury-related deaths in the United States in 1980, 3,313 occurred in children aged 1 to 4 years.

Burns

Burns account for 22% of deaths in this age group, with the highest risk to those under 5. Burns most commonly occur in house fires, then scalds (Table 24-2). Other causes include flames, contact with hot objects, electrical and chemical burns, and ultraviolet radiation. Prevention of house fires may be aided by legislation requiring smoke detectors in all buildings (18).

Adult supervision to prevent severe burns from matches or clothing ignition is essential. Parents and children should be instructed that, if clothing ignites, they should immediately roll on the floor or ground and not run, as running will increase the oxygen feed to the fire and cause more extensive burns. Parents should not purchase loose nightgowns or cotton clothing for their children and check to see if clothes are treated with flame retardants. Cigarettes are a major cause of house fires; the complete lack of legislation

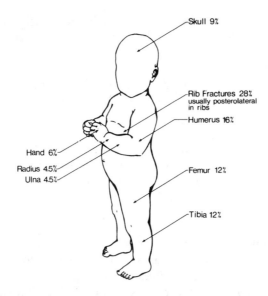

Skull 9%

Rib Fractures 28%
usually posterolateral
in ribs

Humerus 16%

Hand 6%

Radius 4.5%
Ulna 4.5%

Femur 12%

Tibia 12%

Figure 24-1. Skeletal injuries in the battered child: 66% occur in children under 3 years of age, 33% in children under 6 months. Data from a survey of 265 fractures in 74 children (1). (Courtesy of the Ottawa Civic Hospital.)

controlling the slow-burning characteristics of cigarettes contributes to the death toll. Gasoline and other flammable liquids should always be stored in child-proof containers.

About half of all scalds in children under 5 are caused by hot tap water. If the hot-water tank thermostat is set at 120°F, scalds occur after 10 minutes of exposure, at 125°F, after 2 minutes of exposure; and at 130°F, after 30 seconds of exposure. Legislation requiring hot water tanks to have a maximum temperature of 120°F could almost eliminate this source of burns. Adequate supervision of small children is the most significant way to prevent scalds. A

Table 24-2. Burns in children aged 1 to 4

Cause	Preventive strategy	Quality of evidence
House fires	Sprinkler systems	Firm evidence
	Modify burning characteristics of cigarettes	Suggestive evidence
	Smoke detectors	No clear evidence
Clothing ignition	Instruct to roll rather than run if on fire	Suggestive evidence
Scalds	Hot-water heater set at 120° F maximum	Firm evidence
Electrical burns	Extension cords not used	No clear evidence
	Plastic plugs in outlets	Firm evidence
Contact burns	Parental supervision	No clear evidence

change in the design of coffee-makers in Denmark produced FIRM EVI-
DENCE of a two-thirds reduction in burns caused by hot coffee in small children (19).

Electrical burns in 1- to 4-year-olds most commonly occur on the hands,
face, or mouth. Almost all accidents involve electrical extension cords, with
the child's saliva from his or her sucking on the cord conducting the electric-
ity. Plastic plugs to fill empty sockets prevent children's inserting objects into
them.

Contact burns from hot surfaces are best prevented by supervision and
physical protection. Chemical burns from small batteries used in calculators
and radios have become an increasing problem in the last 5 years.

Drowning

Drowning accounts for 21% of injury-related deaths in 1- to 4-year-olds. The
most common sites are pools, streams, or lakes near children's homes. Prevention includes providing toddlers with swimming lessons. There is
SUGGESTIVE EVIDENCE that training 18-month-old children to swim reduces the number of pool accidents by half (20). However, such training does
not substitute for adult supervision. There is FIRM EVIDENCE that legislation requiring pool protection—by 4-foot, 4-inch-high fences with self-lock-
ing gates—has significantly reduced drownings (21, 22).

A very important point to note is that children who have apparently
drowned in very cold water are protected against neurological damage. In a
child whose body temperature has fallen below 32°C, full neurological recov-
ery can occur, with up to 2 ½ hours required to obtain spontaneous pulse and
respiration (23). Victims submerged for up to 40 minutes in cold water have
been resuscitated, whereas 4 to 6 minutes is the usual limit in warm water.

Table 24-3. Deaths from injuries in children aged 1 to 4

Cause	Percent of deaths	Preventive strategy	Quality of evidence
Burns	22	See Table 24-2	
Drowning	21	Fence swimming pools	Firm evidence
Motor vehicle accident	15	Proper restraints	Firm evidence
Pedestrian accident	13	Modify traffic patterns in residential areas	Suggestive evidence
Choking/suffocation	6	Back blow–chest thrust maneuver	No clear evidence
Falls	3	Playground inspection	Firm evidence
Poison	3	Personal counseling	No clear evidence
Other	17		

Motor vehicle accidents

Fifteen percent of deaths in the 1- to 4-year age group occur in motor vehicle accidents. The major factor for reducing this figure is use of adequate in-vehicle restraints. Advocacy for legislative change combined with physicians' emphasis on the importance of using such restraints should improve vehicle safety.

Pedestrian–motor vehicle accidents

Children hit by motor vehicles on roadways account for 13% of deaths in 1 to 4 year olds. There is little a physician can do from his or her office to create a safer environment for children to play in. There is CLEAR EVIDENCE that educational programs for children under age 5 are beneficial. The most significant preventive approach has been noted in Scandinavia, where new housing developments include roadways designed to reduce and slow traffic in pedestrian areas (24).

Choking

Choking and suffocation account for 6% of deaths in this age group. It is important that toys, especially those used by children under 3, have parts larger that 1.24 cm in diameter. Items such as hot dogs, pieces of meat, and peanuts are particularly dangerous in 1- to 4-year-olds. Prevention and handling of choking as outlined for infants less than 1 year old also apply in this age group.

Falls

Falls represent only 3% of deaths from injuries in young children. As children develop and become more active, the incidence of falls climbs steadily, to peak at about 8 years of age. Playground equipment and playground surfaces should be inspected for safety and playground supervisory personnel should be educated in their maintenance. Such personnel should also be educated about proper playground behavior and the public educated about the importance of playground safety. Such a program in one community produced FIRM EVIDENCE of a 22% reduction in injuries (25).

Poisoning

Poisoning accounts for 3% of injury-related deaths but a much higher level of morbidity in this age group. The introduction of child-proof drug containers as well as of child-proof containers for household poisons has significantly reduced poisonings. There is SUGGESTIVE EVIDENCE that a variety of attempts at one-to-one counseling and media campaigns have not significantly reduced the incidence of poisoning (15, 16). The advice for how to prevent these problems is outlined in the section on poisoning in infants, above.

5 TO 14 YEARS

As children become more independent and increasingly mobile, the risk of injuries rises. In this age group in 1980, 5,224 injury-related deaths were recorded, representing 24% of all childhood injury-related deaths (Table 24-4).

Motor vehicle accidents

Twenty-two percent of injury-related deaths in this age group are the result of motor vehicle accidents. Seat-belt laws and parent education about the importance of appropriate restraints for all children in any vehicle is essential. A variety of simple engineering improvements in the roads, such as reducing curves and hills, would significantly decrease mortalities. Also, if rigid structures were not built on or beside highways, highway mortalities would be reduced.

Pedestrian–motor vehicle accidents

Pedestrian injuries account for 19% of the fatal injuries in this age group. They tend to occur between noon and 6 P.M. on urban roads, especially on

Table 24-4. Deaths from injuries in children aged 5 to 14

Cause	Percent of deaths	Prevention strategy	Quality of evidence
Motor vehicle accident	22	Seat belts	Firm evidence
Pedestrian accident (struck by car)	19	School education programs Driver incentives Environmental design	Firm evidence Firm evidence Firm evidence
Drowning	15	Water safety education	No clear evidence
Burns	10	Educational programs	Suggestive evidence
Bicycle accident (struck by car)	7	Helmets Education Regulation enforcement Creation of bicycle lanes	No clear evidence No clear evidence Suggestive evidence Firm evidence
Choking/suffocation	4	Back blow–chest thrust maneuver	No clear evidence
Motorcycle accident (struck by car)	2	Driver education	No clear evidence
Other	21		

through-streets. The lower the speed limit, the less severe are the injuries and the lower is the mortality rate. Thus, the more the urban environment is designed to keep children away from traffic, the lower is the injury rate. The risk of injury decreases steadily from ages 5 to 10, with a 5-year-old boy having six times the risk of being injured that a 10-year-old has (10).

Probably the most instructive finding was made in Alabama, where a Pedestrian Safety Education Program administered to eighteen thousand school children aged 7 to 8 significantly reduced the injury rate (26). Promising drivers rewards such as lowered insurance or tax reductions and threatening those who have accidents with economic penalties have both been demonstrated to reduce pedestrian injuries in children (27, 28).

Drowning

Drowning causes 15% of injury-related deaths in the 5- to 14-year-old age group. Mortality for males is significantly higher than that for females. The most significant intervention is extensive water safety education, such as the program provided through the Red Cross.

Burns

Burns cause about 10% of fatal injuries in this age group. The types of burns differ from those found in the younger age groups. House fires are serious, but the children's mobility somewhat reduces the risk. Fire-setting is at its highest incidence as a behavior problem in 5- to 10-year-old boys. Such behavior usually occurs in curious children who may benefit from educational programs. Pathological fire-setters and their families often require extensive counseling and therapy.

Boys aged 5 to 15 are at risk for gasoline burns. Most often they use gasoline to augment an already active fire or charcoal burner. The explosive flames may ignite the clothing of other children. If the gasoline is used in a basement, the fumes, which are very heavy, stay near the floor and can be explosively ignited by a pilot light or a cigarette.

Fireworks present a particular risk for children in this age group. Many jurisdictions have outlawed them. They should be available to children only under strict supervision.

Bicycle–motor vehicle accidents

Accidents in which a bicycle is struck by an automobile account for 7% of the fatal accidents in this age group. Boys aged 6 to 12 have the highest nonfatal injury rates and boys aged 10 to 14 have the highest fatality rates.

Head injuries are by far the most serious. In Massachusetts the Statewide Childhood Injury Prevention Program found that 20% of injuries involved fractures, 26.8% involved open wounds, 36% involved contusions, and 6.3% involved significant head injuries. Prevention strategies, including the wearing of helmets, have not been demonstrated to reduce the severity of head injuries.

The education of bicycle riders, although it makes the most sense, has not been properly evaluated. The enforcement of bicycle regulations and providing a seminar for those who break the law have been documented to result in a 50 to 100% reduction in accidents, but these results have not been published. Separating bicycle traffic from vehicular traffic has been demonstrated in Scandinavia to reduce morbidity and mortality from bicycle injuries (24).

Choking

Choking causes about 4% of the fatal injuries in children in this age group. Meat, large pieces of food, and other foreign bodies are the objects commonly aspirated. Initial attempts to clear the airway, then four back-blows to the suprascapular area, followed by four chest thrusts using the fingers or palm of the hand constitute the recommended approach to acute choking (see section on choking in infants, above).

Motorcycle accidents

Motorcycle riders struck by cars account for 2% of the fatal injuries in this age group. There is little documentation of these injuries for this age group. Licensing authorities should prevent children in this age group from riding motorcycles.

15 TO 19 YEARS

In the United States in 1980, 12,259 deaths occurred in this age group, representing 55.8% of all injury-related deaths to children (Table 24-5).

Motor vehicle accidents

A shocking 59% of all fatal injuries in this age group occur in the occupants of motor vehicles. The high incidence of motor vehicle accidents among young drivers has long been documented by insurance companies. Males aged 16 to 25 have the highest incidence of fatal motor vehicle accidents of any age-sex group. An attempt to reduce the often fatal combination of alcohol and driving in this age group has been made in Massachusetts and elsewhere where legal drinking age was raised from 19 to 21. Unfortunately, no decline in mortality has occurred (30).

Table 24-5. Deaths from injuries in children aged 15 to 19

Cause	Percent of deaths	Preventive strategy	Quality of evidence
Motor vehicle accident	59	Seat belts	No clear evidence
Drownings	8	Red Cross program	No clear evidence
		Alcohol & drug education	No clear evidence
Motorcycle accident (struck by car)	6	Driver education	No clear evidence
Pedestrian accident (struck by car)	6	School education	Firm evidence
		Driver incentives	Firm evidence
Burns	3	Environmental design	Firm evidence
Poisoning	2	No strategy	
Falls	2	Use of appropriate equipment to prevent sports injuries	Suggestive evidence
Other	14		

The assumption that driver education programs are likely to reduce the incidence of motor vehicle injuries in 16- to 20-year-olds has not been substantiated. Discontinuing school driver education programs in one jurisdiction significantly lowered the mortality in the teen-age group (31). The explanation for this phenomenon was that reducing the number of 16-year-olds starting to drive resulted in fewer accidents. Unfortunately, alcohol is involved in at least one-half of all fatal motor vehicle accidents. At present, there is no known effective strategy to prevent these tragedies.

Drowning

Drowning accounts for 8% of the fatal injuries in this age group. An Australian study found that alcohol or drugs were involved in one-third of drownings (32). Since the highest functions of reasoning and decision making are the first affected by ethanol intake, the equivalent of 3 to 4 pints of beer will dull the senses enough to cause a person who is submerged not to struggle. A combination of water safety practice, swimming instruction, and warnings about the adverse effects of alcohol when swimming is currently the only preventive strategy, but there is NO CLEAR EVIDENCE of its efficacy.

Motorcycle accidents

Motorcycle riders struck by automobiles account for 6% of the fatal injuries in this age group. The patterns and approaches outlined above for bicycle riders are applicable.

Pedestrian–motor vehicle accidents

Pedestrians struck by cars account for 6% of the fatal injuries in this age group; most injuries occur after dark at an intersection. About one-half of the drivers involved in pedestrian accidents were found to be negligent. The discussion of this subject for the 5- to 15-year-old age group applies to the 15- to 19-year-old group as well.

Burns

Burns account for 3% of accidental deaths. Little can be added to the discussions about burns for the previous age groups.

Poisoning

Poisoning accounts for 2% of the fatal accidents in this age group. Drug overdoses in this group must be assessed individually and treated according to the type of drug and dosage. Accidental poisoning may occur in people who transport cocaine by ingesting plastic packages. Each packet contains a fatal dose of cocaine, so, if the packets leak, poisoning results.

Falls

Falls in this age group, usually sports-related, cause 2% of deaths. Other than appropriate head and neck protection in rough sports, no specific strategies in this age group have been proven effective.

Table 24-6 outlines the known beneficial counseling and preventive strategies that have been proven effective (FIRM or SUGGESTIVE EVIDENCE). It summarizes the strategies available to physicians and communities to reduce the very significant death toll of childhood injuries.

Table 24-6. Effective preventive strategies (FIRM EVIDENCE)

Hazard	Positive outcome measures	Reference
Automobile accident	Seat-belt use	33
	Car-seat use	10, 34, 36
Burns	Purchase of smoke detectors	37
	Use of outlet covers	38
	Reduced home hot-water heater setting	39
Falls	Playground assessment of number of falls	40
Poisonings	Possession of ipecac syrup	41, 42
	Knowledge of poison prevention strategies	43

REFERENCES

1. Annual Report of the U.S. National Center for Health Statistics, Bethesda, Maryland. 1982.
2. Greensher, J. *Aspiration Accidents. Handbook on Accident Prevention*. Baltimore, Md.: Harper and Row, 1980, pp. 49–52.
3. Greensher, J., Mofenson, H. Emergency treatment of the choking child. *Pediatrics* 70:110–112, 1982.
4. Gordon, A., Bolton, M., Ridocpho, P. Emergency management of foreign body airway obstruction. In *Advances in Cardiopulmonary Resuscitation*, Safar, P., Exam, J.O., eds. New York: Springer-Verlag, 1977, pp. 39–50.
5. Day, R. Differing opinions on emergency treatment of choking. *Pediatrics* 71:976–977, 1983.
6. Williams, D., Clark, S. The heart saver baby: A CPR course for young parents. *Canada Family Physician* 31:1005–1008, 1985.
7. Baker, S. Motor vehicle occupant deaths in young children. *Pediatrics* 64:860–861, 1979.
8. Reinsinger, K., Williams, A. Evaluation of programs designed to increase protection of infants in cars. *Pediatrics* 62:280–287, 1978.
9. Williams, A., Wells, J. Evaluation of the Rhode Island child restraint law. *Am. J. Public Health* 71:742–743, 1981.
10. Reisinger, K., Williams, A., Wells, J., John, C.E., Roberts, T.R., Podgainy, H.J. Effect of pediatricians' counseling on infant restraint use. *Pediatrics* 67:201–206, 1981.
11. Pearn, J., Brown, J., Wong, R., and Bart R., Bathtub drownings.: Report of 7 cases. *Pediatrics* 64:68–70, 1979.
12. Gallagher, S., Hunter, P., Hatch., E. A home injury prevention program for children. Paper presented at American Public Health Association Annual Meeting, Montreal, 1982.
13. Kravitz, H., Driesung, L., Gomberg, R., et al. Prevention of accidental falls by counselling mothers. *Il. M. J.* 143:570–574, 1973.
14. Chaffe Bahomon, C. Dimensions of pediatric poisoning incidents. *Statewide Childhood Injury Prevention Program Report* Commonwealth of Massachusetts. 1:7–8, 1981.
15. Linyear, A. A systems approach to the prevention and treatment of childhood injuries. Third Year Report of the Bureau of Maternal and Child Health, Richmond, Virginia, 1982.
16. Micik, S., Grossman, K. Childhood accident prevention annual report, July 1, 1981–June 30, 1982. California Children Service Department of Health Services, San Diego.
17. Manoguvrra, A., Krensolk, E. Rapid emisis from high dose ipicac syrup in adults or children intoxicated with anti-emetic or other drug. *Am. Journal of Hospital Pharmacy* 35:1360–1367, 1978.
18. U.S. Fire Administration. *An Ounce of Prevention*. Washington, D.C.: Federal Emergency Management Agency, 1983.
19. Sorenson, B. Prevention of burns and scalds in a developed country. *J. Trauma* 16:249–258, 1976.
20. Whitehead, L., Curtis, L. *How to Watersafe Infants and Toddlers*. Tuscon, Ariz.: H.P. Books, 1983.
21. Pearn, J., Nixon, J. Prevention of childhood drowning accidents. *Med. J. Aust.* 1:616–618, 1977.

22. Pearn, J., Hsia, E. Swimming pool drownings and near drownings involving children. A total population study from Hawaii. *Military Medicine* 190:15–18, 1980.
23. Young, R., Zainoraitis, E., Dooling, E. Neurological outcome in cold water drowning. *J.A.M.A.* 244:1233–1235, 1980.
24. Organization for Economic Cooperation and Development. *Traffic Safety of Children*. Report prepared by an OECD Scientific Expert Group, Paris, 1983.
25. Warner, P. Playground injuries and voluntary product standards for home and public playgrounds. *Pediatrics* 69:18–20, 1982.
26. Howarth, C., Repetto-Wright, R. The measurement of risk and attribution of responsibility for child pedestrian accidents. *Safety Education* 144:10–13, 1978.
27. Furtonbury, J., Brown, D. Problem identification implementation and evaluation of a pedestrian safety program. *Accid. Anal. Prev.* 14:315–322, 1982.
28. Harand, R., Hubert, D. *An Evaluation of California's Good Driver Incentive Program*. Report No. 6. California Division of Highways, Sacramento, 1974.
29. Barmalk, J., Payne, P. The Lakeland accident counter measure experiment. *Proceedings of the Highway Research Board* 40:513–522, 1981.
30. Hingson, R., Morrigan, D., Heeron, T. Effects of Massachusetts raising its legal drinking age from 18 to 20 on deaths from teenage homicide suicide and non-traffic accidents. *Pediatr. Clin. North Am.* 32:221–232, 1985.
31. Robertson, C. Crash involvement of teenaged drivers when driver education is eliminated from high school. *Am. J. Public Health* 70:599–603, 1980.
32. Editorial. Alcohol and drowning. *Med. J. Aust.* 1:157–188, 1981.
33. Bass, L., Thurlow, R. The pediatrician's influence in private practice measured by a controlled seat belt study. *Pediatrics* 33:700–705, 1964.
34. Kanthor, H. Car safety for infants: Effectiveness of prenatal counselling on infant restraint use. *Pediatrics* 58:320–323, 1976.
35. Scherz, R. Restraint systems for the prevention of injury to children in automobile accidents. *Am. J. Public Health* 66: 451–455, 1976.
36. Christophersen, E., Sosland-Edelman, D. An effective hospital-based child passenger safety program. 24th Annual Meeting of the Ambulatory Pediatric Association, 1984. Abstract.
37. Miller, R., Reisinger, K., Blatter, M, et al. Pediatric counselling and subsequent use of smoke detectors. *Am. J. Public Health* 72:392–393, 1982.
38. Dershewitz, R. Will mothers use free household safety devices? *Am. J. Dis. Child.* 133:61, 1979.
39. Thomas, K., Christophersen, E., Hassanein, R. Evaluation of group well-child care for improving burn prevention practices in the home. *Pediatrics* 74:879–882, 1984.
40. Kravits, H., Grove, M. Prevention of accidental falls in infancy by counselling mothers. *I.M.J.* 1:570–573, 1973.
41. Alpert, J., Levine, M., Kosa, J. Public knowledge of ipecac syrup in the management of accidental poisonings. *J. Pediatr.* 71:890–892, 1967.
42. Dershewitz, R., Posner, M., Paichel, W. The effectiveness of health education on home use of ipecac. *Clin. Pediatr.* 22:268–270, 1983.
43. Phillips, W., Little, T. Continuity of care and poisoning prevention education. *Patient Counseling and Health Education* 2:170–173, 1980.

25

PROBLEMS OF ADOLESCENCE

A recent study of a random sample of one thousand adolescents between 12 and 20 years of age revealed that their major health concerns, in rank order, were acne, menstrual problems, nervous and emotional problems, and overweight (1). Teenagers of both sexes were concerned about acne to almost the same degree, whereas emotional problems and concerns about overweight were significantly more prevalent in females. Very few teenagers admitted to problems with drugs, alcohol, or sexual matters. Conversely, public health nurses and school psychologists felt that adolescents' problems with drugs, alcohol, pregnancy, and venereal disease were much more significant (2).

This chapter deals with the major health concerns of adolescents, as well as those problems felt to be significant by school health professionals. Suicide, one of the leading causes of death in adolescents, is discussed in Chapter 23.

ACNE

Prevalence

Almost 50% of adolescents are concerned about acne (1).

Narrowing down and diagnosis

Adolescent acne usually presents no diagnostic problems; the diagnosis is made by visual inspection, and teenagers themselves readily make the diagnosis. Rarely, exposure to certain drugs (systemic or potent topical corticosteroids, or halogens such as the iodides present in certain vitamin-mineral preparations or in "health foods" such as kelp) can cause acne; removal of the exposure usually results in a cure.

The initial lesions of acne are plugs of keratin in the sebaceous follicle lumen. These comedones (blackheads or whiteheads) become inflamed, presumably because normal follicular bacteria cause the plugged-up sebum to break down to fatty acids, which are irritants. Reddish papules, pustules, and cysts then develop. The lesions may occur mainly on the face or develop on the chest, upper back, and shoulders, that is, those sites with high concentrations of sebaceous glands brought to maturity by adolescent surges in androgens. The adolescent with acne will often have a family history positive for acne.

Management of acne

The teenager should be reassured that acne is normal in adolescents and that much can be done to help the condition, although only time will cure it. There is FIRM EVIDENCE that diet does not play a significant role in most cases of acne (3). If an individual teenager notices definite flare-ups every time he or she eats a particular food, and that food is not the only source of an essential nutrient, he or she should avoid it.

There is NO CLEAR EVIDENCE that frequent face washing is any better than ordinary hygiene. Abrasive agents and hexachlorophene are of little benefit. Although there is NO CLEAR EVIDENCE supporting a recommendation to encourage exposure to sunlight, ultraviolet rays seem to improve many patients' condition.

There is FIRM EVIDENCE that topical agents such as benzoyl peroxide in concentrations of 5 to 10% are more effective than placebo (4). Topical retinoic acid has been considered to be an effective agent, but because it causes significant side effects—facial erythema, burning, and dryness—double-blind studies are of questionable value because it is likely that those in the experimental group would have facial redness that would distinguish them from the control group (5). There is SUGGESTIVE EVIDENCE that if benzoyl peroxide, up to 10%, is not effective by itself, the addition of 0.025 to 0.05% retinoic acid, in a cream applied once in the morning and once in the evening will produce results superior to those produced by either agent alone (6). This approach must be used carefully, since both agents can cause facial redness and drying. There is FIRM EVIDENCE that topical tetracycline lotion as well as oral tetracycline are each more effective than placebo (7).

For a patient in the care of a primary care physician, if topical agents alone are not sufficient, a trial of tetracycline or erythromycin, 250 mg four times a day for a few weeks followed by a maintenance daily dose of 250 to 500 mg, should be started. Tetracycline may sensitize the patient to sunlight, and it should not be given to sexually active girls who do not use contraception reliably, since this antibiotic has deleterious effects on the fetus.

For more severe acne that does not respond to this therapy, referral to a dermatologist is indicated. Many such patients will be having difficulty with their self-esteem and normal social interactions. Management of severe multinodular cystic acne, involving dermabrasions, surgical aspiration, and the use of oral retinoic acid, is complex and can produce significant side effects (8).

MENSTRUAL PROBLEMS

Prevalence

Almost one-third of adolescent girls have significant menstrual pain (1). In the past, many girls experiencing dysmenorrhea were thought to be neurotic. Since the role of prostaglandins in producing many of these symptoms has begun to be understood, and since new pharmacologic treatments result in excellent rates of improvement, psychosomatic factors have been deemphasized.

Narrowing down

Primary dysmenorrhea is a disorder that begins 6 to 12 months after menarche: since the first period is anovulatory, and dysmenorrhea occurs only after ovulation, the typical history is one of painless menstruation for the first year. Painful menstruation secondary to pelvic pathology is termed secondary dysmenorrhea. Endometriosis and pelvic inflammatory disease are the major conditions to consider in girls who have pelvic tenderness. A rare cause of cyclic pelvic pain, along with primary amenorrhea, is hematocolpos due to complete obstruction of the lower genital tract.

Diagnosis

The typical patient presents with pain that begins a few hours prior to or concurrent with the menstrual flow. The pain lasts several hours to several days, is colicky and mainly suprapubic, and radiates to the lower back and thighs. There may be gastrointestinal complaints as well as headache. A pelvic examination in sexually active patients will help detect pelvic tenderness and possible endometriosis or pelvic infection. For patients with atypical histories who are virgins or who are difficult to examine, pelvic ultrasound should be ordered.

Treatment of menstrual problems

Analgesics such as acetylsalicylic acid have an effect on prostaglandin synthesis and may be sufficient treatment in girls with mild dysmenorrhea. There is FIRM EVIDENCE that, for more severe symptoms, nonsteroidal antiinflammatory antiprostaglandin agents such as naproxen sodium, 275 mg three or four times per day, are effective (9). If these agents do not control symptoms, ovulation can be inhibited using any of the standard oral contraceptive preparations; this will inhibit the cyclic synthesis and release of prostaglandin and thus relieve dysmenorrhea.

NERVOUS AND EMOTIONAL PROBLEMS

Adolescents tend to have problems with their parents, self-esteem, school performance, and peers, and they worry about their prospects for the future. They are also concerned about their sexuality. In confidential interviews with teenagers, the acronym SIEVE—for sexuality, image, emancipation, vocation, and education—is helpful to remember. Use the third person technique to ask questions: "Some people your age are starting to date—how about you?" or "Some teenagers who are dating have intercourse and are concerned about pregnancy—how about you?" Most teenagers are not offended by this intrusion into their personal lives. Questions such as, "Many teenagers are concerned about their appearance—they're too tall or too fat, or their skin is bad—are you?" will open the door for a teenager to begin discussing some of his or her concerns. To ask about developing autonomy and responsible decision making, questions such as, "Some kids your age have arguments with their parents about bedtimes, homework, etc.—do you?" are effective. Many teenagers who are concerned about their physical attractiveness, for example, acne, will not ask their physicians for help, even though they see the physician for other problems (10).

It is reasonable for a physician to spend a few minutes going through a brief "emotional" questionnaire, using SIEVE, in an attempt to identify problems that the teenager is reluctant to volunteer. SIEVE questions can be asked during visits for other purposes, for instance, camp or school check-ups, or for specific problems such as a rash or sore throat. When teenagers are not troubled in these areas, the questions and answers take only a few minutes. If there are problems identified—difficulties at school, peer pressure about drugs—a return visit can be scheduled specifically to deal with them.

Management of problems identified after SIEVE

Sexuality Concerns about late maturation (small penis, delayed growth spurt in males; small breasts, delayed menarche in girls) can best be dealt with after a careful history and physical examination. It is important for the physician to be familiar with the wide range of normality and Tanner's charts of sexual maturation. These are thoroughly covered in standard pediatric texts. In almost all cases, the teenager will be found to be developing normally; a follow-up visit 6 months later to assess growth velocity in height and weight, and to check again for signs of sexual maturation, will show a normal rate of progress. Delayed maturity in very short girls should provoke particular concern: Turner's syndrome is a distinct possibility.

Teenagers' concerns about masturbation can easily be dealt with by reassuring them that virtually all teenagers engage in this practice; to a greater or lesser degree. Similarly, adolescent males with gynecomastia can usually be reassured that this is a common phenomenon that almost always disappears spontaneously.

Sexually active teenagers of both sexes should be counseled about contraception and venereal disease. There is NO CLEAR EVIDENCE that lecturing teenagers about the risks of sexual intercourse decreases sexual activity; similarly, there is NO CLEAR EVIDENCE that educating teenagers about contraception increases adolescent sexual activity. There is FIRM EVIDENCE that the newer, low-dose contraceptive pills, used appropriately in nonsmoking healthy women under 35 years of age, are remarkably effective and safe.

Image Almost 50% of teenage girls think they are too fat, even though most of them are not (11). Although this is primarily a cultural phenomenon, it is reasonable to ask what a girl concerned about her weight is doing to control her weight. Although there is NO CLEAR EVIDENCE that early detection prevents anorexia nervosa, most clinicians feel that early diagnosis is associated with a better prognosis. The treatment of obesity and anorexia is discussed in Chapter 17. Other growth problems are discussed in Chapter 19.

Emancipation Having determined that an adolescent's parents are having difficulties allowing the teenager to develop responsible decision making, the physician can frequently help by mediating disputes between the patient and the parents. A typical source of friction is the teenager's desire to go out and visit friends before doing his or her homework. If the teenager is doing reasonably well in school, most parents can be made to understand that growing up means choosing priorities, and that most responsible teenagers will do their homework if they are allowed to decide when to do it, since they themselves want to succeed. Allowing increasing decision making does not mean emancipating teenagers completely, since it is their responsibility to continue to do reasonably well in school. If, having been allowed the choice of when to do homework, an adolescent's grades begin to fall, then he or she is not yet mature enough to be allowed that degree of decision making. Mediation can be used in other problems of emancipation, such as choice of friends, clothes, smoking, and drinking.

Vocation Adolescents' answers to questions about their plans for the future are often revealing. Some may show frustration or despair, such as, "Why make plans—we're all going to be blown up anyway." Others may have unrealistic goals, such as a wheelchair-bound 15-year-old boy's wanting to be a race car driver or a high-school student's wanting to be a doctor when she is barely succeeding at school. Although there have been no studies demonstrating the efficacy of physicians' counseling in this area, it is worth exploring the teenager's vocational plans if only to identify unrealistic goals or feelings of depression, and to refer the teenager for vocational, family, or personal counseling. Although it is felt that such counseling may be helpful, there is little evidence to support this view.

Education Performance at school and relationships with teachers and peers are good indicators of how likely a teenager is to achieve the societal goals of success in the work place and in human relations. There are few controlled studies to demonstrate the effectiveness of early identification and remediation of learning, social, or behavior problems in adolescents. Similarly, the role of the primary care physician in managing problems in this area has not been clearly defined. There is FIRM EVIDENCE (12) that parents of a child with learning problems can be taught to improve their child's self-esteem. There are no such studies dealing with teenagers. Even without firm evidence, the burden of suffering of many of these teenagers and their families may be great, and the primary care physician, in collaboration with psychologists and educators, may have an important role to play in alleviating that burden.

PROBLEMS IDENTIFIED AS IMPORTANT BY SCHOOL HEALTH PROFESSIONALS

Drugs and alcohol

Sixteen percent of teenagers use recreational drugs and 52% drink alcoholic beverages (1). Although fewer than 2% of adolescents feel they have problems with drugs or alcohol use, school nurses and psychologists feel that such problems are more prevalent (2). The role of the physician is to determine whether the adolescent is merely experimenting because of peer pressure or does in fact have a problem. If the latter, then a referral to an agency set up to help with these problems or to a private mental health specialist may be indicated. The effectiveness of treatment for drug and/or alcohol problems in adolescents has not been well studied. Preventive interventions in the schools, particularly those involving smoking, show great promise (13).

Pregnancy

In the United States, about 10% of teenage girls become pregnant each year; this rate is at least twice the rate of that in other developed countries. About one-half of the pregnant girls have abortions; the other half give birth and, in most cases, keep their babies (14). About 25% of teenagers aged 13 to 19 years have had sexual intercourse, with about 50% of girls having had intercourse by age 19 (1). Clearly, preventing unwanted pregnancies should be a high priority. The physician now has available the most effective contraceptive ever developed to prescribe to sexually active girls—the low-dose "pill". Since about 85% of teenagers see their doctors each year (10), the physician is able to assess the patient's sexual activity and to advise (males and females) about contraception. In North America, no physician has ever been sued for prescribing oral contraceptives to sexually active minors. In most Western countries it is felt that prescribing contraceptives to minors without parental consent is preferable to unwanted pregnancy.

Some physicians inform all teenage girls in their practices that, although they do not encourage early sexual activity, they will prescribe the pill if it seems likely that the girl will become sexually active. This approach may make it easier for a young woman to speak up who would otherwise be unwilling or embarrassed to ask for contraception before she has intercourse. This might decrease the teenage pregnancy rate because the first few months of intercourse are often the time a girl is most likely to be unprotected against pregnancy.

Venereal disease Symptomatic gonorrhea causes a purulent discharge and burning on urination in both sexes; unfortunately, many girls with gonorrhea are asymptomatic. The organism is fastidious and requires specific transport and culture techniques; laboratories experienced in handling *Neisseria gonorrhoeae* should be consulted. For uncomplicated urethritis or vulvovaginitis, a single intramuscular dose of 4.8 million units of aqueous procaine penicillin plus 1 gram of oral probenecid is recommended by the U.S. Public Health Service. Amoxicillin, 3 grams orally with 1 gram of probenecid, may be used in single-dose therapy. For teenagers who are allergic to penicillin, 500 milligrams of tetracycline orally four times a day for 5 days, may be used; whenever possible, single-dose therapy with penicillin or amoxicillin is preferred because lack of compliance with the tetracycline regimen may be a problem. Patients with gonorrhea should have a serologic test for syphilis upon diagnosis and again 3 months later.

Chlamydia causes approximately 40% of cases of nongonococcal urethritis. The offspring of infected mothers are at risk of neonatal conjunctivitis and infantile chlamydial pneumonia. If this diagnosis is suspected, the microbiology laboratory should be consulted for advice about techniques and media for the transport of specimens. Erythromycin, 1 gram daily for 14 days, will eradicate the organism.

REFERENCES

1. Feldman, W., Hodgson, C., Corber, S., Quinn, A. Health concerns and health-related behaviours of adolescents. *Can. Med. Assoc. J.* 134:489–493, 1986.
2. Hodgson, C., Feldman, W., Corber, S., Quinn, A. Adolescent health heeds, III: Perspectives of health professionals. *Can. J. Public Health* 76:167–170, 1985.
3. Fulton, J.E., Plewig, G., Kligman, A.M. Effect of chocolate on acne vulgaris. *J.A.M.A.* 210:2071–2074, 1969.
4. Ede, M. A double-blind comparative study of benzoyl peroxide, benxoyl peroxide-chlorhydroxygunoline, benzoyl peroxide-chlorhydroxyquinoline-hydrocortisone, and placebo lotions in acne. *Curr. Ther. Res.* 15:624–629, 1973.
5. Kligman, A.M., Mills, O.H. Pseudofolliculitis of the beard and topically applied tretinoin. *Arch. Dermatol.* 107:551–552, 1973.
6. Hurwitz, S. The combined effect of vitamin A acid and benzoyl peroxide in the treatment of acne. *Cutis* 17:585–590, 1976.
7. Blaney, P.J., Cook, C.H. Topical use of tetracycline in the treatment of acne. *Arch. Dermatol.* 112:971–973, 1976.
8. Haber, R.M. The management of acne vulgaris—Part III. *Modern Medicine of Canada* 39:1325–1331, 1984.
9. Lundstrom, V. Treatment of primary dysmenorrhea with prostaglandin synthetase inhibitors—A promising therapeutic alternative. *Acta. Obstet. Gynecol. Scand.* 57:421–428, 1978.
10. Hodgson, C., Feldman, W., Corber, S., Quinn, A. Adolescent health needs, II: Utilization by adolescents of health services. *Adolescence* 21:383–390, 1986.
11. Feldman, W., McGrath, P., O'Shaughnesy, M. Adolescent's pursuit of thinness. *A.J.D.C.* 140:294, 1986.
12. Mahoney, W., Kuzzell, N. Roche, D., Feldman, W. Sustained beneficial effect of a parenting course for parents of children with learning disabilities. *Clin. Invest. Med.* 8:A175, 1985 (Abstract).
13. Flay, B.R., D'Avernas, J.R., Best, J.A., Kersell, M.W., Ryan, K.B. Cigarette smoking: Why young people do it and ways of preventing it. In *Pediatric and Adolescent Behavioral Medicine*, McGrath, P., Firestone, P., eds. New York: Springer, 1983, pp. 132–183.
14. Alan Guttmacher Institute. 360 Park Avenue South, New York, New York 10010. *Report to the Ford Foundation on the Findings and Policy Implications of a Comparative Study of Teenage Pregnancy and Fertility in Developed Countries.* 1985.

26

COPING WITH STRESS

This chapter focuses on the effects of stressful situations and how families cope with them. Stress can be acute or chronic: Acute stress refers to a difficult event whose impact is relatively short in duration, for example, short-term parental unemployment, marital discord, brief hospitalization of a child or parent, financial setback, or change of school. Chronic stress refers to events whose sequelae last over a long period. Examples include the birth of a child who is handicapped or chronically ill, and the loss of a parent to death or through divorce. Chronic stress may begin with short-term stress, and short-term stress may be superimposed on background chronic stress.

The advantage of examining stress in a noncategorical fashion, rather than looking at each kind of stress individually, is that even though there are a limitless number of potential stressors, there are a limited number of strategies that can be used to assist families in dealing with them. Moreover, the response to the stressor may be determined by the family and their situation more than by the exact nature of the stressor.

PREVALENCE

The prevalence of acute stress is not well documented, in part because of the difficulty of defining what constitutes acute stress. However, substantial numbers of families experience acute stress in any given month. Coddington (1) found that the average annual number of stressful life events experienced by children in a year was 3.67. Roghmann and Haggerty (2) found that on any given day there was a 30% chance of a family's experiencing an episode of stress.

The prevalence of chronic stress can be estimated by examining the rates of specific stressors. For example, approximately 1 in 10 children has a chronic illness (3); approximately 1 in 3 children born in the 1970s will experience the divorce of their parents (4); and levels of unemployment in many areas in North America are above 20%.

NARROWING DOWN

Narrowing down the problem of stress consists of delineating the sources of stress, the effects of the stress, and the resources available to the family to assist them in coping. *The most important factor is the physician's being attuned to the lives of his or her patients, being aware enough to ask the right questions and to listen to patients' concerns.* With chronic stress there are predictable times when the stress may be exacerbated. For example, families with developmentally delayed children are likely to have minicrises when the child should be beginning to walk but does not, when the child begins school, and when the child reaches puberty. Similarly, in families that have lost a loved one, the anniversaries of the loss and holidays may be particularly stressful. In many instances, the narrowing down process is especially helpful for the family. With the help of a concerned physician, they may begin to be able to understand what they are experiencing and to see their reactions as normal responses to difficult situations.

While some events are likely to be stressful for most people, an individual's perception of a particular event plays a major role in the amount of stress he or she feels. Indeed, a blessed event in one family, such as a birth of a female child, may be construed as a tragedy in another family. Temperament, culture, and the presence of other stresses influence an individual's approach to specific events.

Sources of stress

The sources of stress are extremely varied. Coddington (1), in his life events scales, lists between thirty and forty stressors for each of four age groups. For children, the major sources of stress are family, school, and peers. Parents are likely to experience stress from marital, work, and personal problems, as well as from the medical and behavioral problems of their children. Social isolation and lack of family support can be sources of stress in and of themselves, as well as potentiating factors in all other forms of stress. Drug abuse, alcoholism, and familial mental illness frequently are major stressors. The ill health of a family member, particularly a parent or a child, can produce major stress, and the cost of health care is frequently an additional stress in chronic illness. Poverty, crime, and the fear of crime are major sources of stress for many families.

Effects of stress

Acute stress, even of a minor nature, substantially increases one's chances of becoming ill (2). Physical symptoms in the child or parent may include pain, anorexia, fatigue, and sleep problems. Psychologic reactions may include depression, anxiety, children's noncompliance with adults' requests, and short temper. Children's language and social and self-care behavior may regress. In addition, parents may become more rigid and controlling of their children, which results in behavior reactions in the children (5). Self-medication or alcohol abuse by parents may exacerbate the symptoms of stress. Both denial and overreaction may occur. A higher than typical level of these types of difficulties in a family should prompt the physician to inquire about current levels of stress and coping abilities.

Certain types of chronic stress, such as the birth of a physically or mentally handicapped child, may lead to "chronic sorrow," a long lasting feeling of pain or dysphoria that never disappears and surfaces during other crises. Chronic sorrow is not an abnormal or neurotic response but a realistic response to tragedy. Chronic sorrow occurs in approximately three-quarters of parents with disabled children (6, 7). Although divorce rates are not higher among families with chronically ill children, marital distress does appear to be more prevalent (8).

Children with chronic illness are at risk for psychological problems, but it is important to realize that the majority of children with chronic disease adapt very well (1, 9). Children with sensory problems and children with low self-esteem may be most vulnerable (3).

Poverty, a major source of chronic stress, is associated with a higher risk of both behavioral and medical problems (10). Hospitalization because of illness or surgery, with the attendant separation from family, is stressful for many children and may result in behavioral regression.

Coping resources

Coping resources affect how families and children react to stress. The most important resources available to families and children under stress are personal resources, family resources, and community resources. Personal coping resources include the intellectual, emotional, physical, and financial competencies of the individual child and parents. Family coping resources include the resources of the extended family (grandparents, aunts, uncles, cousins, and friends) available to the family and child. Community coping resources include government and public services, private agencies, volunteer agencies, and religious institutions. Such agencies include a wide range of health and social services, such as hospitals, clinics, visiting homemakers, nursing and therapy services, financial services, food services, specialized and general play and activities services, Big Brothers and Sisters, day-care centers, nurseries, and other schools.

MANAGEMENT OF STRESS

There are five major strategies that the primary care physician can use to assist families coping with acute or chronic stress:

1. Identification of the role of stress.
2. Clinical intervention.
3. Supportive counseling.
4. Comprehensive case management.
5. Advocacy.

Identification

Many people having difficulty coping with stress are unaware that they are under stress; however, identification of the problem is often very helpful. In some cases, this insight alone will allow them to help themselves reduce the number of stressful situations that they find themselves in and mobilize their resources to cope.

Clinical intervention

The most common clinical intervention for stress undertaken by a primary care physician will either involve symptomatic medical treatment of the symptom (such as sleep disorder or headache) or medical treatment of the underlying problem causing the stress. However, for some patients and some primary care physicians, psychologically oriented interventions such as various forms of stress management, relaxation training (11), clinical hypnosis (12), preparation for aversive events (13), or family or individual therapy may be appropriate. With trained practitioners, there is SUGGESTIVE EVIDENCE that each of these methods may be effective in combating the effects of stress in some circumstances. In many situations, no clinical intervention is possible. Life-style changes, including more nutritious diet, more exercise, and smoking cessation, will probably do no harm if approached sensibly. However, there is NO CLEAR EVIDENCE that they will enhance the individual's ability to deal with stress.

Supportive counseling

Parents and children generally view their own physicians as wise and dedicated professionals who can help them. Consequently, in times of stress, the wise counsel of a person who is aware of the medical and social aspects of a family's situation may prove invaluable. The aim of supportive counseling is not to treat psychological problems but to provide understanding and assistance to families who are having a difficult time and to reduce the probability of problems developing within the family. The major components of supportive counseling are empathic listening, commonsense problem solving, and encouragement.

Self-help groups that are organized by lay persons and that may rely on some professional input often provide a form of supportive counseling that may be as helpful as professional supportive counseling. Self-help groups are most frequently organized around specific disease or clinical conditions, such as the Association for Children with Learning Disabilities, the Epilepsy

Association, and the Cystic Fibrosis Association. The local public library can provide information about the local branches of various groups.

There is SUGGESTIVE EVIDENCE of the effectiveness of supportive counseling for families of chronically ill children (14), and graduates of Neonatal Intensive Care (15).

Frequently, parents under stress consult their physician because of regressive behaviors in their child, such as secondary enuresis, infantile speech in a child who knows how to talk, or temper tantrums that previously were resolved. After carefully listening to what the concerns are, the physician combines reassurance that such regressions are normal and transient with specific suggestions about how to manage the behaviors. The importance of giving a little more affection or attention to the child should be emphasized.

Problem solving will often involve helping families to discern the exact nature of their difficulty, the resources that are available to them, and how to make contact with those services. To do this, the primary care physician must not only know the families but also have knowledge of the available community resources.

Comprehensive case management

For families with a chronically ill child, one of the most frustrating ordeals is having to deal with several different specialists. An important role for the primary care physician in such a case is to ensure that comprehensive care is given; with many specialists the child and family may seem to get lost in the process of diagnosis and treatment (3). There is SUGGESTIVE EVIDENCE that such a role may be helpful to families (14).

Advocacy

There are two different forms of advocacy: social or institutional advocacy, in which social or political change is sought to alleviate conditions that cause stress or disease (16, 17), and individual advocacy, in which the needs of specific patients are championed in an institutional forum. There is FIRM EVIDENCE that institutional advocacy can work in some situations if the advocates are persistent and well-organized (17). Similarly, it is clear that a physician who has marshaled his or her facts and is firmly committed to helping a particular family can often obtain a more appropriate school placement or a speedier passage through the bureaucratic jungle (18).

REFERENCES

1. Coddington, R.D. The significance of life events as etiologic factors in the diseases of children, II: A study of a normal population. *J. Psychosom. Res.* 16:7–18, 1972.

2. Roghmann, K.J., Haggerty, R.J. Daily stress, illness, and the use of health services in young families. *Pediatr. Res.* 7:520–526, 1973.
3. Pless, I.B. Effects of chronic illness on adjustment: Clinical implications. In *Advances in Behavioral Medicine for Children and Adolescents*, Firestone, P., McGrath, P., Feldman, W., eds. Hillsdale, N.J.: Lawrence Erlbaum Associates, 1983, pp. 1–21.
4. Wallerstein, J. Separation, divorce and remarriage. In *Developmental-Behavioral Pediatrics*, Levine, M.D., Carey, W.B., Crocker, A.C., Gross R.T., eds. Philadelphia: W.B. Saunders, 1983, pp. 241–255.
5. Mash, E.J. Families with problem children. In *Children in Families Under Stress. New Directions for Child Development*, No. 24. Doyle, A., Moskowitz, D.S., eds. San Francisco: Jossey-Bass, 1984, pp. 65–84.
6. Wikler, L., Wascow, M., Hatfield, E. Chronic sorrow revisited: Parent vs. professional depiction of the adjustment of parents of mentally retarded children. *Am. J. Orthopsychiatry* 51:63–70, 1981.
7. Olshansky, S. Chronic sorrow: A response to having a mentally defective child. *Social Casework* 43:190–193, 1962.
8. Sabbeth, B.F., Leventhal, J.M. Marital adjustment to chronic childhood illness: A critique of the literature. *Pediatrics* 73:126–131, 1984.
9. Kellerman, J., Zelter, L., Ellenberg, L., Dash, J., Rigler, D. Psychological effects of illness in adolescence. I. Anxiety, self esteem, and perception of control. *J. Pediatr.* 97:126–131, 1980.
10. Select panel for the promotion of child health. *Better Health for Our Children: A National Strategy*, vols. 1–3. Washington D.C.: U.S. Department of Health and Human Services, 1981.
11. Cautela, J., Groden, J. *Relaxation: A Comprehensive Manual for Adults, Children and Children with Special Needs.* Champaign, Ill.: Research Press, 1978.
12. Hilgard J.R., LeBaron, S. *Hypnotherapy of Pain in Children with Cancer.* Los Altos, Calif.: Kaufman, 1984.
13. Melamed, B.G., Siegel, L.J. *Behavioral Medicine: Practical Applications in Health Care.* New York: Springer, 1980.
14. Stein, R.E.K., Jessop D.J. Does pediatric home care make a difference for children with chronic illness? Findings from the Pediatric Ambulatory Care treatment study. *Pediatrics* 73:845–853, 1984.
15. Perrault, C., Coates, A.L., Collinge, J., Pless, I.B., Outerbridge, E.W. Family support system in newborn medicine: Does it work? Follow-up study of infants at risk. *J. Pediatr.* 108:1025–1030, 1986.
16. Berger, L.R. The pediatrician's role in child advocacy advances. *Pediatrics* 29:273–291, 1982.
17. Micik, S.H., Alpert, J.J. The pediatrician as advocate. *Pediatr. Clin. North Am.* 31:243–249, 1985.
18. Battle, C.U. The role of the pediatrician as ombudsman in the health care of the young handicapped child. *Pediatrics* 50:916–922, 1972.

27

HOSPITALIZATION OF INFANTS AND CHILDREN

This chapter deals with the indications for hospitalizing infants and children, problems associated with hospitalization, ways of preventing these problems, and alternatives to hospitalization. In two separate studies (1, 2), pediatricians arrived at a consensus of the indications for hospitalization:

1. Extensive diagnostic procedures, such as 24-hour urine collections in infants or renal biopsy.
2. Acute medical or surgical illnesses requiring frequent nursing, medical, or paramedical care, such as measuring vital signs more than three times per day, loss of consciousness, need for intravenous fluids or medication, oxygen therapy, and/or suction, or surgery that cannot be done on an out-patient basis.
3. Patients referred from other regions where specialized medical care is not available.
4. Social reasons, for example, the assessment of an infant for possibly nonorganic failure to thrive.

In both studies, in two separate communities, approximately 40% of children were judged to have been hospitalized inappropriately.

Aside from the cost of the hospital care of infants and children, which is usually higher than that for adults because of the need for a higher staff/patient ratio, there are other important reasons for taking care that hospitalization is necessary, as discussed below.

PSYCHOLOGICAL EFFECTS

There is FIRM EVIDENCE (3) that the hospitalization of preschool-aged children results in anxiety and regressive behavior, including disturbances of feeding, toilet training, and sleeping, that persist for as long as 3 months after hospitalization. These disturbances were found to be much less frequent and less prolonged in an experimental group of hospitalized children whose parents were allowed increased visiting time, who became ambulatory early in their hospital stay, who participated in a special play program, who underwent psychological preparation for and support during painful procedures, and whose parents received preparation training in assisting their child before and during the hospitalization. Other studies (4, 5) have shown that the single most distressing event for a hospitalized child is diagnostic venipuncture.

HOSPITAL-ACQUIRED INFECTIONS

During the respiratory syncytial virus season, one-third of hospitalized infants were infected while in the hospital, and all who were infected became ill, showing respiratory symptoms and signs, regardless of the original reason for their admission (6). The stay of infants who acquired the infection in the hospital was extended by 12 days more than would be expected for their admission diagnosis. In addition to the morbidity and financial costs, infants and children who acquire infections in the hospital are usually isolated, which diminishes their contact with adults and other children and adds to the psychological burden of the hospitalization. Other viruses, such as rotavirus, are significant causes of hospital-acquired infections.

FLUID AND ELECTROLYTE PROBLEMS WITH INTRAVENOUS THERAPY

Whenever possible, infants and children should be encouraged to take fluids and nutrition orally, since their own thirst and hunger can usually define their needs more sensitively than can the most knowledgeable physician. In addition, most foods taken by mouth in the hospital contain the necessary nutrients in the proportions that can be handled by a child's gastrointestinal and renal systems. The three most common problems associated with intravenous fluid therapy (when it is truly required) are the following.

Inappropriate electrolyte solution

There are almost no indications for the administration of intravenous dextrose and water without electrolytes. Although there are no prevalence data available, the authors are aware of deaths and permanent brain damage that have occured in rural hospitals where physicians have prescribed dextrose and water without electrolytes. Brain swelling, brain damage, coning, and death may occur. For most purposes (e.g., diarrhea and vomiting so severe that oral rehydration is unsuccessful—very rare—or respiratory distress so severe that drinking is difficult—also rare), a solution of one-third normal saline in 5% glucose with added potassium, 25 to 30 mEq/L, is satisfactory. For some reason, physicians often forget that potassium is an essential electrolyte. As soon as it is clear that the patient is not in acute renal failure, that is, he or she *is* producing urine, potassium must be added to the fluid, or else hypokalemia, with disastrous effects on skeletal and heart muscle, may develop, possibly with a fatal outcome.

Inappropriate volumes of fluid

There are a number of formulae based on weight or surface area that can be used to calculate the maintenance fluid requirements. The formula used to calculate oral fluid requirements in gastroenteritis (see Chapter 5) can also be used to calculate intravenous fluid requirements. This formula is effective in maintenance therapy and has the advantage of being simple: $[100 - 3 \times age (years)]$ ml/kg/24 hours. Thus, for a 4-year-old child weighing 20 kilograms, the maintenance fluid level would be $100 - 12 = 88 \times 20 = 1,760$ ml/24 hours, which can be rounded off to 1,800 ml/24 hours = 75 ml/hour. For mild dehydration, add 25 ml/kg/24 hours; for moderate to severe dehydration, add 50 to 75 ml/kg/24 hours. As mentioned earlier, each infant and child is different, and the best initial calculations cannot replace repeated clinical assessments to ensure that the volume and composition of the intravenous fluids are appropriate and still required.

Excessive duration of intravenous feeding

No prevalence data are available, but the authors have seen numerous examples of malnutrition, including protein-calorie malnutrition, resulting from intravenous fluid therapy being extended too long. It is important to remember that as soon as the infant or child is able to take fluids and nutrition orally, they should be given them, since the combination of a normal diet, intestinal absorption, and renal function produces a much more satisfactory result than can an intravenous regimen. The case in which oral nutrition cannot be given within hours to several days of the start of intravenous feeding is extremely unusual. Should this occur, a consultation is in order. If the physician works in a remote rural hospital, the child should be transported to the nearest center where specialist care is available.

ALTERNATIVES TO HOSPITALIZATION

Alternatives to hospitalization, even for the indications listed at the beginning of the chapter, should always be considered. For example, extensive diagnostic procedures such as 24-hour urine collection in infants are usually not necessary. If one should be necessary, and if the parents can stay home with the child and be properly instructed, urine collection bags can be used at home. Other collections, such as 72-hour stool collections for fat determination, can be reliably collected by parents.

Acute medical or surgical illness may also be amenable to home care. For example, the loss of consciousness such as occurs in a febrile seizure is not per se an indication for hospitalization. In fact, if the diagnosis is certain and the parents can be successfully reassured of the benign nature of this problem, the child can be sent home as soon as he or she is awake, alert, and responsive.

The third indication for hospitalization mentioned at the start of the chapter, a referral from an area where specialized care is not available, is not likely to be seen in a primary care practice. In many tertiary care settings, a referral of this type is no longer an indication for hospitalization, since motel-type facilities are frequently nearby and the child can receive ambulatory care in a specialized setting for diagnosis, treatment, or both.

The fourth indication for hospitalization, a social reason, is clearly appropriate in many situations, for example, assessing the condition of an infant who may be suffering from environmental deprivation. However, hospitalization for social reasons is sometimes abused. For example, the hospitalization of a child who could otherwise be investigated and treated as an outpatient but whose parents are both working, may not be appropriate.

The long-term hospitalization of a child with severe chronic or terminal illness is, fortunately, rare. Although such children have significant medical and nursing needs, many hospitals and communities are developing home-care and school-care programs that enable these children to remain in the community as long as possible. Some children's families may also avoid the child's hospitalization in the terminal states of disease and decide to let death occur at home.

REFERENCES

1. Feldman, W., Duggan, C. Unnecessary hospitalization of infants and children. Proceedings of the Canadian Pediatric Society Annual Meeting, Kingston, Ontario, June 13, 1971 (Abstract).
2. Duff, R.S., Cook, C.D., Wanerka, G.R., Rowe, D.S., Dolan, T.F. Utilization review of pediatric inpatient care. *Pediatrics* 49:169–173, 1972.
3. Prugh, D.G., Staub, E.M., Sands, H.H., Kirschbaum, R.M., Lenihan, E.A. A study of the emotional reactions of children and families to hospitalization and illness. *Am. J. Orthopsychiatry* 23:70–106, 1953.
4. Burling, K.A., Collipp, P.J. Emotional responses of hospitalized children: Results of a pulse monitor study. *Clin. Pediatr.* 8:641–646, 1969.
5. Sheridan, M.S. Children's feelings about the hospital. *Soc. Work Health Care* 1:65–70, 1975.
6. Hall, C.B., Douglas, R.G., Geiman, J.M., Messner, M.K. Nosocomial respiratory syncytial virus infections. *N. Engl. J. Med.* 293:1343–1346, 1975.

28

PROBLEMS OF PATIENT COMPLIANCE

Compliance, in the medical setting, is "the extent to which a person's behavior (in terms of taking medications, following diets, or executing lifestyle changes) coincides with medical or health advice" (1). Noncompliance is the failure to follow medical or health advice. Three types of noncompliance can present problems for the primary care physician working with children: nonattendance at scheduled appointments, failure to take medication as prescribed, and failure to change behavior as suggested. However, noncompliance should be considered a problem only if it interferes with the therapeutic efficacy of the suggested advice.

Some noncompliance may be harmless, and in some cases noncompliance may be therapeutic. For example parents who reduce their asthmatic child's theophylline medication from what was prescribed in order to balance the control of symptoms against side effects may be appropriately titrating the dose (2); this should not be considered to be a compliance problem. Similarly, the diabetic adolescent who does not take a second injection of insulin as prescribed but maintains his or her single daily dosage because it is more acceptable to him or her represents a compliance problem only if the disease is out of control.

PREVALENCE

The prevalence of noncompliance varies with the definition of noncompliance and the regimen prescribed. Noncompliance in terms of children's missing medical appointments ranges from 19% (3) to 52% (4). Noncompliance with a medication regimen in acute conditions ranges from 42 to 82% (5). In chronic conditions, noncompliance has been measured to be 12 to 89% (5). Noncompliance with recommendations to change behavior is also high. For example, approximately 70 to 75% of recommendations to use seat belts are not complied with (6). Compliance with suggestions to change parents' behavior in order to influence their child's behavior is also low, but the exact prevalence is unknown.

APPOINTMENT-KEEPING

Narrowing down

Noncompliance in the form of missing appointments requires a system for tracking missed appointments. Some missed appointments may not be a problem, but failure to attend appointments for immunization, suspected child abuse, growth problems, and diabetes is important, and a method for identifying these missed appointments should be devised.

Management of noncompliance with appointment-keeping

There is FIRM EVIDENCE that the most cost-effective method of improving appointment-keeping for immunizations is mailing reminders that are specific as to what is required (7). A similar system for other important missed appointments is likely to be effective.

MEDICATION AND ADVICE

Narrowing down

Although blood and urine measurements are the most sophisticated methods of determining noncompliance with medication regimens, they are rarely necessary in primary care. The easiest method of determining compliance with a medication regimen or advice is to ask the adolescent patient or parent. Such questions as, "How many days this week did Jimmy get both doses of medication?" or "How many days did you spend special time with Jimmy?" These are preferable to general questions, such as, "Is Jimmy getting his medication?" or "Did you spend time with Jimmy?" A second method is to ask the parents to record medication consumption or following advice in a diary. Global physician judgment as to who is compliant is not accurate (FIRM EVIDENCE) (5).

Management of noncompliance with medication and advice

There are at least two prospective ways of attempting to reduce noncompliance: reducing the impediments to compliance, and identifying potential noncompliers and targeting these individuals for intensive efforts to

Table 28-1. Approach to compliance in children's health care

Is compliance important in this case?

If not, then implement routine procedures.

If so, then ask the patient about possible difficulties with regimen and solve each problem individually.

increase their compliance. Impediments to compliance include the patient's inability to perceive the benefit of the regimen, the cost of the regimen, its clarity, complexity, or convenience, and a lack of supervision or built-in reminders. Reducing these barriers, as outlined in Table 28-2 is likely to lead to improved compliance (SUGGESTIVE EVIDENCE) (5, 8).

Noncompliers may be prospectively identified by asking the adolescent patient or parent "Are you the type of person who might have trouble keeping this appointment schedule/taking this medication regularly/following these suggestions?" or, "What types of problems might come up in keeping this appointment/taking this medication/following this advice?" (9). Subsequent to identifying the patients at high risk for noncompliance, the physician should make an intensive effort to overcome obstacles to compliance or to tailor the regimen to the needs of the family.

Directly teaching the child (even the preschool-aged child) to follow the regimen may, in some situations, be an effective adjunct to instructing the parents (10). The use of peer models may be effective in increasing compliance in adolescents (11).

Table 28-2. Barriers to compliance in children's health care

Barrier	Example	Problem-solving technique
Lack of perceived benefit	Patient stops taking antibiotic when earache seems to be gone	Warn: "Take drug until all is gone" and explain reason
Cost	Expensive antibiotic prescribed	Assess cost of drug for family; use least expensive alternative
Lack of clarity	Vague instructions "Take 1 tablespoon"	Write down instructions Prescribe "standard spoonful"
Complexity	Multiple medications with multiple schedules	Simplify regimen; arrange home care supervision
Convenience	t.i.d. dosage	b.i.d. or single-doses; suggest pill box
Side effects	Nausea, diarrhea	Warn about side effects; suggest management

REFERENCES

1. Haynes, R.B. Introduction. In *Compliance in Health Care*, Haynes, R.B., Taylor, D.W., Sackett, D.L., eds. Baltimore: Johns Hopkins University Press, 1979, pp. 1–2.
2. Deaton, A.V. Adaptive noncompliance in pediatric asthma: The parent as expert. *J. Pediatr. Psychol.* 10:1–14, 1985.
3. Alpert, J. Broken appointments. *Pediatrics* 34:127–132, 1964.
4. Nazarian, L.F., Mechaber, J., Charney, E., Coulter, M.P. Effects of mailed appointment reminders on appointment keeping. *Pediatrics* 53:349–352, 1974.
5. Dunbar, J. Compliance in pediatric populations: A review. In *Pediatric and Adolescent Behavioral Medicine: Issues in Treatment*, McGrath, P.J., Firestone, P., eds. New York: Springer, 1983.
6. Miller, J.R., Pless, I.B. Child automobile restraints: Evaluation of health education. *Pediatrics* 59:907–911, 1977.
7. Yokely, J.M., Glenwick, D.S. Increasing the immunization of preschool children: An evaluation of applied community interventions. *J. Appl. Behav. Anal.* 17:313–325, 1984.
8. Masek, B.J., Jankel, W.R. Therapeutic adherence. In *Behavioral Pediatrics: Research and Practice*, Russo, D.C., Varni, J.W., eds. New York: Plenum, 1982.
9. Litt, I.F. Know thyself—Adolescents' self-assessment of compliance behavior. *Pediatrics* 75:693–696, 1985.
10. Chang, A., Dillman, A.S., Leonard, E., English, P. Teaching car passenger safety to preschool children. *Pediatrics* 76:425–428, 1985.
11. Jay, M.S., DuRant, R.H., Shoffitt, T., Linder, C.W., Litt, I.F. Effect of peer counselors on adolescent compliance in use of oral contraceptives. *Pediatrics* 73:126–131, 1984.

INDEX